Study Guide for CANPC™ Exam

Fully Compliant with 2022 Code Books

Compliant with the 2022 codebooks ICD-10-CM, CPT, HCPCS II and 2022 ASA Crosswalk(R), and 2022 Relative Value Guide(R).

CANPC Essentials for Accurate and Efficient Medical Coding for Anesthesia and Pain Management

Extensive Study Guide for Preparation for CANPC™ – Certified Anesthesia and Pain Management Coder Examination 2nd Version

A Refresher Training Manual for Practicing Anesthesiology and Pain Management Coders

Vino C. Mody Jr., Lic., COC, CPC, CCS, CCS-P, CMC, CANPC, CCVTC, CEDC, COPC, CNPR

 The book is compliant with the 2022 codebooks ICD-10-CM, CPT, HCPCS II and 2022 ASA Crosswalk(R), and 2022 Relative Value Guide(R).

First Printing: January 2022

ISBN: 978-1-947333-06-2

Suwanee Press
1115 River Laurel Dr.
Suwanee, Georgia, 30024

Dedicated to

My parents, my brother, and my uncle Dr. Manoj Shah (a practicing OBG and former president of AMA, Georgia Chapter) for their support and encouragement

Table of Contents

Acknowledgements

I would like to express my gratitude to several individuals within healthcare institutions and the local chapter of the American Academy of Professional Coders (AAPC) in El Paso, Texas for their guidance and opportunities provided for learning, teaching, and networking with healthcare professionals in Texas. My sincere thanks to Yesenia Ceniceros, an instructor, and supervisor at Southwest University; Ms. Ellen Eastman, President of AAPC Local Chapter; Ms. Carrol Kozerinsky, President of AAPC Local Chapter; and Roberta Pell, organizer of Local Chapter events and proctor for examinations for various healthcare related certifications. I learned a lot from the teaching sessions I conducted and presentations by administrative professionals at the local chapter and institutes. I appreciate the guidance I received from my employers, Tara Broadie, Manager of the Medical Administration team at HGS USA Company, and Kathleen Cahill, CEO of Mesa Hills Specialty Hospital in El Paso, medical administrative functions. I wish to offer special thanks to my father, Vino Mody, for his excellent help with the editing of this book and for coordinating with the designer and publisher to get the book ready for production.

Preface

This book presents and elaborates on fundamental principles of anesthesiology coding and how to approach anesthesia and pain management coding accurately and efficiently. The book covers key steps for anesthesiology coding and a correct method for determining the overall anesthesiology code for each case. Included in the book are a variety of useful topics: unit calculations, anesthesia and pain management modifiers, physical status qualifying circumstances—or what I call emergency conditions, and clinical viewpoints for each case. The presentation is concisely written to get the point across in a meaningful way, and it is easy to understand and explain. The book comprises 71 cases, including a 15-question Certified Anesthesia and Pain Management Coder (CANPC™) simulation exam and 56 cases discussed to teach proper anesthesiology coding techniques. Pain management cases are also outlined. The examples are based on material from a few excellent sources, such as AHA Coding Clinic subscriptions, AAPC CANPC™ study guides, and the Optum General Surgery workbook.

The book is a clear guide for people who would like to learn anesthesiology coding or refresh their skills. The book is structured as a tutorial and will be a useful study guide in your employee training programs for Anesthesiology and Pain Management coding.

The best and proven successful approach to becoming well-versed in medical coding is to learn the basic concept of coding and medical terminology and, last but not least, to practice. My recommendation is that you read the introduction and then complete cases 16 through 71 first, followed by the CANPC™ simulation exam (cases 1 to 15). The CANPC™ simulation exam is based on my recollection of the actual American Academy of Professional Coders (AAPC) exam, which I passed.

The CANPC™ examination is challenging and requires substantial preparation. Anesthesiology involves complex terminology that you must learn, apart from the coding techniques. In fact, your coding speed and precision would depend on your understanding of anesthesia terminology, which you can learn from several affordable sources. A Glossary of Anesthesia and related terminology by Sanford L. Klein is a useful and comprehensive guide that you might consider including in the literature that will help you prepare for the CANPC™ exam and a career in Anesthesiology coding. The American Society of Anesthesia Technologists and Technicians also offers magazines and lectures you may wish to look into for useful sources. The local chapter of the AAPC nearest to your town may hold talks by Anesthesiology and Pain Management experts that you should consider attending.

The Book Outline

The aim of this book is to instruct the reader on the most appropriate approaches to anesthesiology and pain management coding. It is aimed at coders, billers, and other healthcare workers who are preparing to take the Certified Anesthesia and Pain Management Coder (CANPC™) examination. Its goal is to present concepts and applications that will aid in passing the exam while providing insights into the multitude of scenarios that coders face when presented with actual coding cases. The book also provides clinical viewpoints (*from a physician's perspective*) to explain the rationale underlying different coding decisions. The various cases presented in the book highlight the correct coding method and provide practice in applying coding principles.

The author provides a formal calculation method for determining overall anesthesia coding. His formula can be universally applied by all coders, and involves the following steps:

1. Determining the appropriate anesthesia code for surgical procedures provided, using the ASA Crosswalk Lookup.

2. Assigning modifiers to identify the anesthesia provider.

3. Reporting physical status modifiers for anesthesia services.

4. Reporting qualifying patient circumstance codes when appropriate.

The author describes key concepts that the coder needs to understand, such as field avoidance and special positioning of the patient, as these change the coding. He then presents a formula that can be used to determine the "units" (base, time, physical status, and emergency units) that, when added together, give a total "unit for anesthesia services" that can then be used to generate the required medical code.

The method used to arrive at the code involves the use of the ASA Crosswalk® and evaluation of the base value units for each procedure performed, the type of anesthesia used, and the extent of patient pre-, peri-, and postoperative procedures. Variations include obstetric anesthesia; management of epidurals; trigger point, sacroiliac, and facet joint injections; discography; the use of pain pumps; nerve blocks; and the use of neurolytic agents.

Case Studies: The 71 case studies presented in the book are designed to simulate the CANPC™ examination. They provide the reader with practice to facilitate passing the exam and becoming a faster and more effective coder. The first fifteen cases are an actual simulation of the exam; the remaining cases provide extra practice in coding. Examples of case studies are the following:

Case 1: Involves placement of arterial, central venous, and Swan Ganz catheters under general endotracheal anesthesia in a 71-year-old male with multiple health issues. The use of the ASA crosswalk lookup and the universal formula developed by the author gives a total unit code of 41.0, based on the base units, the time, the physical status of the elderly patient, and the emergency nature of the procedure. The overall code is 00541-AA-P3, +99100, 36620, 36556, 93503. The clinical rationale behind this final code is discussed.

Case 19: Involves general endotracheal anesthesia in a 65-year-old woman undergoing cataract surgery. Here, the ASA crosswalk lookup and the total units for this type of eye surgery on this age of patient generate the overall code of 00142-AA, P1. Again, a discussion is provided for the clinical rationale by which the code was derived.

Case 20: Involves general endotracheal anesthesia in a 75-year-old patient with bladder cancer. The overall code is 00912-AA-P3, based on the procedure itself, the presence of cancer, and the age of the patient (over seventy years). The further discussion provides the clinical rationale for the final code.

Introduction

This book covers anesthesiology and pain management coding to generate the correct overall anesthesiology code for each case. The purpose of the book is to help coders, billers, and other workers in healthcare organizations prepare for the Certified Anesthesia and Pain Management Coder (CANPC™) examination. While this book will serve as a great aid to get you ready for the exam, it may not replace years of your experience performing the coding function in anesthesiology and pain management medical practice. Learning concepts and applications by practicing on a large number of exercises—as included in books like this and written by subject matter experts—is necessary if you are to attain the necessary speed and accuracy in the coding process. However, the ultimate source of this knowledge, speed, and accuracy is actual experience working in diverse situations under the guidance of experienced mentors. The material presented can also be used to provide training to coding students and workers employed in pain management coding. Clinical viewpoints (*from a physician's perspective*) are offered throughout the book as appropriate, and these cover the rationale for the cases discussed. The book will also be useful to professionals taking coding certification examinations conducted by AAPC and AHIMA. The first 15 cases highlight principles outlined in the Study Guide for CANPC™ 2014/2016 for full anesthesiology coding according to the American Academy of Professional Coders.

Medical diagnosis and treatment procedures are involved, and they demand experience and expertise in proper and prompt coding to obtain rapid payment approval for procedures and the services delivered to patients. Getting CANPC™ certification adds to your credentials and credibility when working with billers and insurance companies, and it ultimately helps your employer, whether a private medical practice or a hospital. The AAPC and AHIMA membership extends your contacts with coding practitioners and supports your credibility as a professional coder.

Relevant topics of diagnostic coding for anesthesiology and pain management are reviewed in the book. As a prerequisite to passing the CANPC™ examination, you must know how to identify the appropriate ICD-10-CM codes and the right sequencing of diagnostic codes, particularly when multiple codes are required to assess the actual disease condition. An ASA Crosswalk®, Relative Value Guide®, and an audit worksheet are permitted for reference during the CANPC™ examination.

This book will help you prepare for the CANPC™ exam, in conjunction with the literature available in Study Guide for CANPC™ 2016 and 2021; these will help you to get ready for the exam. The discussion provided for every case highlights the correct method for anesthesiology coding, thereby enhancing your chance for success on the CANPC™ exam by American Academy of Professional Coders. The material presented also helps you as a coder in your ability to do accurate work by giving you additional practice and apply the coding principles to actual cases. The exercises are structured for beginners to advanced level practitioners. Knowing the details and excellent points regarding how to perform anesthesiology coding is imperative for passing the exam. After rigorous practice of the principles discussed in this book, you should be able to come up with the correct codes by following the instructions provided. (For the exam, MD means the medical doctor and CRNA means certified registered nurse anesthetist. Pain management coding is also covered.)

(For the CANPC™ exam, if you code for a different CPT answer, still perform the ASA Crosswalk Lookup on your selected CPT codes and use the universally applied method in the same way to determine the overall anesthesiology code for the case. This suggestion will help you identify the anesthesiology code correctly.)

CPT Coding

CPT coding discipline requires that you follow a structured process. Anesthesiology coding is not straightforward and requires attention to detail. I have developed a universally applied formal method for determining the overall anesthesia code for a case. The following are my recommended steps for anesthesia coding I encourage you to follow:

<u>Step 1: Determine the appropriate anesthesia code for the surgical procedures provided, utilizing the ASA Crosswalk Lookup</u>

For example, the corresponding anesthesia code for CPT code 66984 is Extracapsular cataract removal with insertion of intraocular lens prosthesis (1 stage procedure), manual or mechanical technique is 00142 Anesthesia for procedures on the eye; lens surgery. CPT code=base value units= (corresponding) anesthesia code; 66984=4 base value units=00142

The method for anesthesiology coding is outlined later in this book, under that title.

For two or more CPT codes, select the overall anesthesia code with the highest base value units. For a tie, select the anesthesia code that corresponds to the first-listed CPT code.

<u>Step 2: Assign modifiers to identify the anesthesia provider</u>

The modifiers for the provider can be either for the anesthesiologist (or doctor) or for the CRNA(s). Distinguishing between an Anesthesiologist or Doctor and CRNA modifier codes is important. Anesthesiologist or Doctor codes are for the billing anesthesiologist, whereas CRNA codes are for the billing CRNA.

See the table in HCPCS II.

- AA [Anesthesiologist] Anesthesia services performed personally by an anesthesiologist
- AD [Anesthesiologist] Medical supervision by a physician; more than four concurrent anesthesia procedures [more than 4 CRNAs is included here]
- QK [Doctor] Medical direction of two, three, or four concurrent anesthesia procedures involving qualified individuals [2, 3, or 4 CRNAs is included here]
- QS Monitored anesthesia care (MAC) service
- QX [CRNA] CRNA service: with medical direction by a physician
- QY [Doctor] Medical direction of one certified registered nurse anesthetist (CRNA) by an anesthesiologist
- QZ [CRNA] CRNA service: without medical direction by a physician

- G8 Monitored anesthesia care (MAC) for deep complex, complicated, or markedly invasive surgical procedures
- G9 Monitored anesthesia care for patient who has history of severe cardio-pulmonary condition
- GC These services have been performed by a resident under the direction of a teaching physician

Step 3: Report physical status modifiers for anesthesia services

PS I through PS VI can be found in the Relative Value Guide®. The base units for each physical status are important in the unit calculation for PS or physical status. PS with corresponding base unit values are listed.

- P1: A normal healthy patient= 0
- P2: A patient with mild systemic disease= 0
- P3: A patient with severe systemic disease= 1
- P4: A patient with severe systemic disease that is a constant threat to life= 2
- P5: A moribund patient who is not expected to survive without the operation= 3
- P6: A declared brain-dead patient whose organs are being removed for donor purposes= 0

Step 4: Report qualifying circumstance codes when appropriate

I call qualifying circumstances codes by the heading Emergency.

Qualifying circumstances with base unit values

- +99100: Anesthesia for a patient of extreme age, younger than 1 year and older than 70= 1
- +99116: Anesthesia complicated by utilization of total body hypothermia= 5
- +99135: Anesthesia complicated by utilization of controlled hypotension= 5
- +99140: Anesthesia complicated by emergency conditions= 2

Field avoidance and special positioning with base unit values

“Field avoidance” means the anesthesia provider does not have access to the patient’s airway during surgery. Any procedure around the head, neck, or shoulder girdle that requires field avoidance, or any procedure requiring a position other than supine or lithotomy, has a minimum base unit value of 5, regardless of any lesser base value assigned to such a procedure in the body of the Relative Value Guide®.

Code additional procedures performed by the anesthesia provider. To count as a separately reportable code on the anesthesiology service, note that the anesthesia provider has to perform the additional procedures, not the surgeon.

To be clear, the following procedures are separately reported for the anesthesiology service if performed by the anesthesiology provider (Anesthesiologist or Doctor or CRNA)

- Insertion of central venous catheters: 36555 or 36556
- Insertion of arterial catheters: 36620 or 36625
- Insertion of Swan Ganz catheter: 93503
- Transesophageal echocardiogram (TEE): 93312

<u>Determine the total units for anesthesia services</u>

For unit calculations, you can use:

- Units = Base + Time + PS + Emergency

Base units (for the anesthesia code), time units (anesthesia time/15), PS (physical status modifier) units, and Emergency (Qualifying circumstances) units are added together to generate the total units.

- Medicare units = Base + Time (For a Medicare patient)

Method for anesthesiology coding

The method for determining the overall anesthesiology code for a case is structured and universally applicable. The method involves utilization of the ASA Crosswalk® and looking at the base value units for each procedure.

Anesthesiology coding

To determine the overall anesthesia code for a case, look up each CPT code in the ASA (American Society of Anesthesiologists) Crosswalk and note the corresponding anesthesiology code with its base unit value. Note that the anesthesiology code with the highest base unit value is the overall anesthesia code for the case for all CPT procedures.

Example:

Anesthesia services provided by an anesthesiologist (PS III)

Arstasis: Introduce access device for self-sealing arteriotomy; Enlarged aneurysm area near the anastomosis to the brachial artery, excise the AV fistula

CPT and ICD-10-CM codes:

- 35011, 35206, 37607, I71.2

Corresponding anesthesia codes with base unit values and CPT codes

ASA Crosswalk Lookup

- 35011 = 10 base value units = 01652
- 35206 = 4 base value units = 01782
- 37607=6 base value units = 01840

In order to select the overall anesthesia code for this case, choose the anesthesia code with the highest base value units; note that the first listed code splits a tie.

- 01652-AA-P3

Types of anesthesia

Several types of anesthesia are available, depending on how deep the anesthesia for the case should be and whether the anesthesia involves the entire body, a region, or only a small area.

Local

- Local anesthesia is bundled with the minor surgery CPT code

Monitored anesthesia care (MAC)

- Deep sedation, in which the patient can respond to painful stimuli but maintains control of the airway

Regional

- Epidurals and nerve blocks
- Provides anesthesia for a region of the body

General

- The patient is unconscious and has no control of the airway

Services included in the anesthesia code for general anesthesia, MAC, or regional anesthesia

The following services are included:

- Pre-operative visits, post-operative visits, patient care during the procedure, administration of fluids and blood, EKGs, temperature measurement, blood pressures, intubation, laryngoscopy, the introduction of a needle or catheter, venipuncture, blood transfusions, blood sample procurement through an existing line, temporary transcutaneous pacemakers, and injections of diagnostic or therapeutic substances.

Obstetric anesthesia

Obstetric anesthesia is anesthesia provided during labor and delivery for a woman. When selecting a code for obstetric anesthesia, check to see if the patient had received neuraxial labor analgesia prior to delivery for pain control and anesthesia. Report 01967 for neuraxial labor analgesia/anesthesia for planned vaginal delivery, including any repeat subarachnoid needle placement and drug injection as well as any necessary replacement of an epidural catheter during labor.

Daily Hospital Management of an Epidural

Daily hospital management of an epidural is reported starting with the first postoperative day (01996) and not on the day of the epidural or subarachnoid catheter placement.

Trigger point injections

In a trigger point injection, a local anesthetic is injected into a trigger point to relieve pain in a muscle. It is counted based on the number of muscles injected, not the number of injections (20552)).

Sacroiliac injection

Sacroiliac injection of anesthetic or steroid utilizing CT or fluoroscopy imaging guidance is included in 27096.

Discography

Discography is performed to see if a disc is the source of a patient's pain. Contrast is injected into the disc, and the patient's response to the injection is documented. Discography (62290 or 62291) combined with radiological supervision and interpretation (72285 or 72295) is performed with contrast injected into the disc.

Epidurals

- Single injection not via indwelling catheter (coded 62310 or 62311)
- Injection, including catheter placement, for continuous infusion of intermittent bolus (coded 62318 or 62319)
- When the epidural is the method for the anesthesia, code the appropriate anesthesia (coded 00100–01999)

Transforaminal epidural

CPT codes are based on the number of levels and regions of the spine and are performed for diagnostic and therapeutic purposes.

- The procedure (64479 -64484) can identify which nerve is causing the pain, and it can be performed for chronic pain.
- If the provider performs ultrasound guidance, code Category III codes as 0228T or 0229T; 0230T, or 0231T.

Pain pumps

Procedures for pain pumps used for pain management or spasticity treatment are reported with codes 62350–62370.

When an intrathecal or epidural catheter is connected to an implantable reservoir or an implantable infusion pump (IIP), codes 62350 or 62351 are reported.

Programmable infusion pumps (PIIP) and IIPs are important for drug delivery systems and for the treatment of a wide range of clinical conditions, such as cancer and chronic pain.

Facet joint injections

Facet joint injections temporarily relieve pain by filling the facet joint with an anesthetic medication that numbs the facet joint and the ligaments and joint capsule that surround the facet joint.

Facet joint injections are used for injections of diagnostic or therapeutic agents in paravertebral facet (zygapophyseal) joints (or nerves innervating that joint) with image guidance (fluoroscopy or CT); these are coded by 64490, 64491, 64492, 64493, 64494, or 64495, depending on the level of the injection. (For example, 64490 is used for cervical or thoracic; single level.)

Nerve blocks

A nerve block is an injection of an anesthetic agent directly (64400–64455) near a nerve to stop pain. When a nerve block is performed for regional anesthesia, report the appropriate anesthesia code (00100–01999).

Destruction by a neurolytic agent

- Neurolytic agents destroy nerve tissue (64600–64640) for ongoing relief of pain for weeks or up to a year due to disease or other abnormality of the nerve root. This procedure is known as a rhizotomy.

Relative value order

CPT codes should be arranged in relative value order, a concept applied in Certified Cardiovascular and Thoracic Surgery Coder (CCVTC) theory. Each CPT code has a relative value unit, as found in the 2022 National Physician Fee Schedule Relative Value File January Release, copyrighted in 2021 by the American Medical Association and in 2022/23 by the American Dental Association. The first-listed CPT code is the CPT code with the highest corresponding relative value unit, followed by the second-listed CPT code, which has the second highest relative value unit, and correspondingly in the same fashion to the last-listed CPT code, which has the lowest relative value unit. All CPT codes in this book are arranged in the correct relative value order, which is important for solving a split-tie in cases of anesthesia coding. In a case of a split-tie in anesthesia coding, the first-listed CPT code in the split-tie is the overall anesthesia code for the case in most cases.

Method for determining the anesthesia code for a split-tie

There is an actual method for determining the anesthesia code for a split-tie not based on relative value order. The split tie occurs when there is a tie of the highest base unit value determined from procedure codes using the ASA Crosswalk. If there are at least two different anesthesia codes linked to the tied highest base value units, the situation is called a split tie. The actual method is that the longer or longest procedure wins the split tie. The anesthesia code which wins the split tie is the overall anesthesiology code for the case. How does one determine which procedure is the longest? The number of lines in the operative report may help one determine which procedure is the longest. For example, the procedure described by more lines in the operative report wins the split tie in terms of anesthesia coding.

Cases for CANPC™ exam simulation

Discussed in the following are case numbers 1 through 71, which the readers need to practice and learn to prepare for the CANPC™ examination and to be better coders. Cases 1 through 15 are a CANPC™ simulation exam, which can help prepare candidates for the actual CANPC™ exam. The candidate should prepare for the CANPC™ exam by first studying AAPC's CANPC™ study guide and then taking the CANPC™ simulation exam (cases 1–15) outlined in this book. The CANPC™ simulation exam in this book is based on the actual exam, and it covers novel material not found elsewhere. Cases 16–71 might be studied first for better learning and application of the method of anesthesiology coding before taking the CANPC™ simulation exam.

Case 1: Thoracotomy

- Anesthesia time: 08:00 A.M. to 2:00 P.M.
- Dr. SC, MD, anesthesiologist, performed the anesthesiology procedure for the case
- A right radial arterial catheter, central venous catheter, and Swan Ganz catheter were placed by Dr. SC at the beginning of the case
- Anesthesiologist performed general endotracheal anesthesia
- PS III
- Pt. is a 71-year-old male with multiple medical problems, COPD, hypertension, hypercholesterolemia, and type 2 diabetes mellitus, who suffered from difficulty in breathing
- Diagnosis: Chronic pneumothorax
- Procedures: Surgical thoracoscopy with therapeutic wedge resection and mechanical pleurodesis

Codes

J93.81, J44.9, E78.5, I10, E11.9, 32666, 32650

Pleurodesis is the surgical fusion of the pleura.

ASA Crosswalk Lookup; CPT Code = Base value units = Anesthesiology code

32666 =15 base value units = 00541

32650 = 12 base value units = 00540

Overall anesthesiology code for the case

00541-AA-P3, +99100

36620, 36556, 93503

00541-AA = Anesthesia for thoracotomy procedures involving lungs, pleura, diaphragm, and mediastinum (including surgical thoracoscopy), utilizing 1 lung ventilation

00541 anesthesiology code has higher base value units than 00540

- AA Anesthesiologist performed the anesthesia for the case
- PS3 = Physical status modifier III
- +99100 Anesthesia for patients of extreme age, younger than 1 year and older than 70
- Since Dr. SC, the anesthesiologist placed the right radial arterial catheter at the beginning of the case, the procedure ~~code~~ for the arterial catheterization is coded separately

- Since Dr. SC, the anesthesiologist placed the central venous catheter at the beginning of the case, the code for the central venous catheterization is coded separately
- Since Dr. SC, the anesthesiologist placed the Swan Ganz catheter at the beginning of the case, the code for the placement of the Swan Ganz catheter is coded separately

Total units = Base + time + PS + Emergency = 15+24.0+1+1=41.0

Case 2: Integumentary system

- Anesthesia time: 09:00 A.M. to 1:20 P.M.
- Dr. DM, MD anesthesiologist performed anesthesiology for the case supervising 1 CRNA
- CRNA service: JS
- Anesthesiologist placed central venous catheter and Swan Ganz catheter
- Anesthesia: General endotracheal
- Anesthesiologist noted emergency condition: bleeding during surgery
- Pt. is a 20-year-old female with no medical problems
- PS I
- Diagnosis: Partial amputation of left middle finger cutting across the finger in an edger in a garden
- Procedures:
- Full thickness graft with the closure of donor site, hand, 2.0 cm X 2.0 cm
- Adjacent tissue transfer, left hand, defect 0.5 cm X 0.5 cm
- Excisional debridement of skin and subcutaneous tissues of the left middle finger

Codes

S68.623A, W29.3XXA, Y92.007, Y93.H2, Y99.9, 15240, 14040-51, F2, 11010-F2-51

ASA Crosswalk lookup

15240=5 base value units=00300

14040=5 base value units=00300

11010=3 base value units=00400

Overall anesthesia code for the case for the billing anesthesiologist

00300-QY-P1 +99140,

36556, 93503

00300 has the highest base unit value

For a tie of the highest base unit value, the anesthesia code corresponds to the first-listed CPT code for the case. In this case, both anesthesia codes are the same for the highest base value units. The first-listed CPT code can be determined from a Relative value file. The CPT code with the highest relative value units is the first-listed code. The first-listed CPT code is 15240.

QY the anesthesiologist directed one CRNA; this is an anesthesiologist's code

P1 - The patient is a normal healthy patient

Overall anesthesia code for the case for the billing CRNA

00300-QX-P1, +99140

Total Units=Base + Time + PS + Emergency = 5 +17.3 + 0 + 2 = 24.3 (Can round up or down)

If the patient were a Medicare patient,

Medicare Total Units = Base + Time = 5 + 17.3 = 22.3

Case 3: Arthroscopic on hip joint

- Anesthesia time 07:45 A.M to 11:00 A.M.
- Anesthesiologist, DD, MD medically directing two CRNAs
- CRNAs, JM, PS
- Anesthesia: Monitored anesthesia care (MAC)
- PS III
- 60-year-old female with pain in right hip while walking. Pain on movement of the right hip.
- Diagnoses: Osteoarthritis of the right hip, chondrocalcinosis of right hip, articular cartilage disorder of right hip
- Procedures: Surgical arthroscopy of hip with debridement/shaving of articular cartilage; resection of labrum of right hip

Codes:

M16.11, M11.251, M24.151, 29862-RT

ASA Crosswalk Lookup:

29862=4 base value units=01202

There is only one anesthesia code for the case. Overall anesthesia code for billing anesthesiologist

01202-QK-QS, P3

QS Monitored anesthesia care (MAC) is the anesthesia provided for this case. MAC involves the patient's ability to control his airway unlike general anesthesia but heavily sedated.

QK Medical direction of two, three, or four (CRNAs) concurrent anesthesia procedures involving qualified individuals.

QK, like QY, AA, and AD are doctor's codes from HCPCS II.

The physical status modifier is P3, a patient with severe systemic disease

Overall anesthesia code for CRNA service

01202-QX-QS, P3

QX CRNA service: with medical direction by a physician (can be for more than one CRNA).

For CRNA's billing code, only choose from QX or QZ.

Units calculation: Time units calculation is Time (in minutes)/15

Units= Base + time + PS + Emergency = 4 + 13.0 + 1 + 0 = 18.0

Case 4: Intracranial

- Anesthesia time: 2:27 P.M. to 8:03 P.M.
- Anesthesiologist, DD, MD directed the anesthesiology for the case
- The neurosurgeon placed a radial arterial catheter, central venous internal jugular catheter, and Swan Ganz catheter
- A cardiologist performed the transesophageal echocardiogram (TEE)
- Anesthesia: General endotracheal
- PS V
- Patient is a 60-year-old patient with uncontrolled hypertension who presents with hypertensive intracerebral hemorrhage and subdural hematoma as shown on CT scan
- Diagnosis: Hypertensive nontraumatic acute subdural hemorrhage; intracranial intracerebral hemorrhage, intraventricular
- Procedure: Burr hole with evacuation and drainage of subdural hematoma

Codes

I62.01, I61.5, I10, 61154-50

Discussion:

Although most acute subdural hemorrhages are the result of trauma, non-traumatic subdural hematomas can result in death. In this case, the patient had both hypertensive intracerebral hemorrhage and subdural hematoma. Neurosurgery was performed to evacuate and drain the subdural hematoma with a burr hole. This case falls into both pain management and anesthesiology

ASA Crosswalk Lookup

61154=9 base value units=00214

Overall anesthesiology code for the case

00214-AA-P5

The anesthesiologist personally provided the general anesthesia for the case.

The radial arterial catheter, central venous internal jugular catheter, and Swan Ganz catheter were placed by the neurosurgeon. For an anesthesiology case, these codes only count if the catheters are placed by the anesthesiologist or CRNA. Therefore, these are not coded. Likewise, the cardiologist performed the TEE. These were important for the case, but the TEE is not also coded for in anesthesiology. Note that the radial arterial catheter, central venous internal jugular, Swan Ganz catheter, and transesophageal echocardiogram are the only separately reportable procedure codes for anesthesiology if placed by the anesthesiologist or CRNA.

This patient is a moribund patient not expected to survive without the operation.

Therefore, the Physical Status modifier is P5.

Units=Base + Time + PS + Emergency =

Time units =336/15 = 22.4

9 + 22.4 + 3 + 0 = 34.4 (round up or down)

Case 5: Open or surgical on humeral head and neck

- Anesthesia time: 06:00 A.M. to 8:17 A.M.
- 2 CRNAs, KR, BQ performed the anesthesia for the case without medical direction by an anesthesiologist
- Anesthesia: General endotracheal
- PS I
- The anesthesia was complicated by utilization of total body hypothermia.
- 50-year-old male with right shoulder pain. He lifts weights regularly. Limited ROM of right arm and pain on movement.
- Diagnosis: Complete rotator cuff tear of right shoulder, not specified as traumatic
- Procedure: Surgical arthroscopy of right shoulder, extensive debridement

Codes

M75.121, X50.0XXA, Y93.B3, Y93.79, Y99.8, 29823-RT

ASA Crosswalk lookup

29823=5 base value units=01630

Overall anesthesiology code for the case for CRNAs

01630-QZ-P1,

+99135

Anesthesia for open or surgical arthroscopic procedures on knee joint

QZ CRNAs performed the service without medical direction by a physician.

P1 the patient is a normal healthy patient.

Total units = Base + time + PS + Emergency = 5 + 9.13 + 0 + 5 = 19.1

The anesthesia was complicated by the utilization of total body hypothermia. Therefore, 5 base value units are assigned from Emergency. The patient is a normal healthy patient; therefore, the physical status modifier is P1.

Case 6: Transurethral (including urethrocystoscopy)

- Anesthesia time: 04:44 P.M. to 05:29 P.M.
- Anesthesiologist KS, MD, performed anesthesiology for the case personally while medically directing five CRNAs
- CRNAs JK, MF, LT, VB, SD
- Anesthesia: General endotracheal
- PS III
- Diagnosis: Patient has a two-year history of vesicoureteral-reflux. Patient has current urinary tract infection. A cystogram is performed, finding a stricture in the urethra
- Procedure: Cystourethroscopy, with calibration and/or dilation of urethral stricture; Injection procedure for cystography

Codes

N13.70, N39.0, B96.89, 52281, 51600-59

ASA Crosswalk Lookup

52281=3 base value units=00910

51600=3 base value units=00910

Overall anesthesiology code for the case

00910-AD-P3

00910 Anesthesia for transurethral procedures (including urethrocystoscopy)

In this case, there is a tie for anesthesia codes. However, the base value units are the same and the corresponding anesthesia code is the same for each CPT code for the case. The first listed code is 52281 with the corresponding anesthesia code 00910. In this case, 52281's corresponding anesthesia code should be used to break the tie as it is the first-listed code. For the Relative value order, 52281 is the first-listed code with 4.41 Relative value units and 51600 is the second-listed code with 1.28 Relative value units.

AD Medical supervision by a physician; more than four concurrent anesthesia procedures

P3 A patient with severe systemic disease; a two-year history of vesicoureteral-reflux and a current urinary tract infection is a severe systemic disease

Overall CRNAs code for the case

00910-QX-P3

QX CRNA service under medical direction by a physician, the anesthesiologist

Total units = Base + Time + PS + Emergency = 3 +3.0 + 1 + 0 = 7.0

Case 7: Intraperitoneal in the lower abdomen

This case will help with the CANPC^{TM} anesthesiology and pain management examination

- Anesthesia time: 11:00 A.M. to 1:03 P.M.
- Anesthesiologist JR, MD personally provided the anesthesiology for the case
- Anesthesia: General endotracheal
- The anesthesia was complicated by emergency conditions.
- PS III
- The patient is a 40-year-old female with perforation of the intestine. She underwent an exploratory laparotomy last week. The patient presented to the E.R. with extreme abdominal pain and tenderness and the patient made an unplanned return to the operating room during the postoperative period. The patient was found to have an emergency bleeding perforation of the intestine.
- Diagnosis: Perforation of the intestine; Other complications of surgical and medical care
- Procedure: Re-opening of recent laparotomy

CPT codes

K63.1, K91.62, 49002-78

Modifier 78=Unplanned return to the operating room during the postoperative period

ASA Crosswalk Lookup

49002=6 base value units=00840

Overall anesthesiology code for the case for the billing anesthesiologist

00840-AA-P3,

+99140

00840 Anesthesia for intraperitoneal procedures in lower abdomen including laparoscopy; not otherwise specified

P3 - The patient has a severe systemic disease, perforation of the intestine

99140 Anesthesia complicated by emergency conditions (specify) (List separately in addition to code for primary anesthesia procedure)

Units calculation

Units = Base + Time + PS + Emergency = 6 + 8.2 + 1 + 2 = 17.2 (Can round up or down for CANPC exam)

Clinical viewpoint

The anesthesia was complicated by emergency conditions manifest by intra-operative emergency bleeding.

Case 8: Lumbar region

- Anesthesia time: 06:00 A.M. to 11:56 A.M.
- Anesthesiologist FR, MD provided the anesthesiology for the case
- Anesthesiologist performed a transesophageal echocardiogram prior to the beginning of the operations.
- Anesthesia: General endotracheal
- PS I
- The patient is a 35-year-old male with severe lower back pains after an auto accident 2 months ago. He has a herniated spinal disk at L5-S1 and spondylolisthesis according to MRI.
- Combined posterior technique with posterior interbody and lateral fusions with decompression, involving a complete laminectomy and bilateral foraminotomies, at L5-S1 is reported using the following codes to Medicare (note that other codes, such as those for instrumentation and bone grafts, may be separately reported):
- Diagnoses: Intervertebral disc displacement; spondylolisthesis
- Procedures: Complete laminectomy and bilateral foraminotomies L5-S1; Combined posterior interbody and lateral fusions with decompression

Codes

M51.26, M43.16, V89.2XXD, Y93.89, Y92.411, Y99.9, 22633, 63047-59

Clinical viewpoint

This case is both anesthesiology and pain management. In this case, the patient suffers from intervertebral disc displacement combined with spondylolisthesis, when one vertebra slips out of place to the vertebra below.

22633 Arthrodesis, combined posterior or posterolateral technique with posterior interbody technique including laminectomy and/or discectomy sufficient to prepare interspace (other than for decompression), single interspace, and segment; lumbar

63047 Laminectomy, facetectomy, and foraminotomy (unilateral or bilateral with decompression of spinal cord, cauda equine and/or nerve root(s), [e.g. Spinal or lateral recess stenosis], single vertebral segment, lumbar

ASA Crosswalk Lookup

22633=8 base value units=00630

63047=8 base value units=00630

Overall anesthesiology code for the case

00630-AA-P1,

93312

00630 Anesthesia for procedures in the lumbar region, not otherwise specified

P1 Other than for the auto accident, the patient was a normal healthy patient with no systemic disease

Units calculation

Units = Base + Time + PS + Emergency = 8 + 23.7 + 0 + 0 = 31.7 (Can round up or down)

Clinical viewpoint

This patient suffered from an intervertebral disc displacement and spondylolisthesis which required two major pain management surgeries. Proper anesthesiology management and pain management were in addition critical to the case. In this case, the correct Relative value order is 22633 followed by 63047. The anesthesiologist performed a transesophageal echocardiogram at the beginning of the case. Therefore, TEE is coded separately. For TEE to be coded separately, the anesthesiologist must perform the procedure.

Case 9: Integumentary system, muscles, and nerves of the head, neck, and posterior trunk

- Anesthesia time: 10:00 A.M. to 11:57 A.M.
- JN, MD anesthesiologist performed the anesthesia for the case
- JS, CRNA helped to perform the anesthesia under the direction of the anesthesiologist
- JS, CRNA placed a radial arterial catheter at the beginning of the case
- Anesthesia: General endotracheal
- PS I
- A 16-year-old boy is brought in because of a skateboarding accident. He sustained open wounds on both lower legs. The surgeon takes the patient to the OR for debridement. The wound on the left leg is 4 cm x 6 cm. The surgeon irrigates the wound and debrides the subcutaneous tissue and skin. When all of the debris is removed, he applies a dressing and then addresses the right leg. The wound on the right leg is 3 cm x 5 cm. This wound is deeper than the last and requires debridement of nonviable muscle, subcutaneous tissue, and skin. What is the proper code selection?
- Diagnoses: Open wounds on lower legs; 4 cm X 6 cm left leg; and 3 cm X 5 cm right leg
- Procedures: Debridement, subcutaneous tissue (includes epidermis and dermis, if performed); first 20 sq. cm or less; each additional 20 sq. cm or part thereof (List separately in addition to code for primary procedure); Debridement, muscle and/or fascia (includes epidermis, dermis, and subcutaneous tissue, if performed); first 20 sq. cm or less

Codes

S81.801A, S81.802A, V00.138A, Y93.51, Y92.480, Y99.8, 11043, 11042, 11045

ASA Crosswalk Lookup

11042=3 base value units=00400

11043=5 base value units=00300

11045=not a primary procedure code

Overall anesthesiology code for the case for the billing anesthesiologist

00300-QY-P1

Overall anesthesiology code for the case for the billing CRNA

00300-QX-P1,

36620

00300 Anesthesia for all procedures on the integumentary system, muscles, and nerves of the head, neck, and posterior trunk, not otherwise specified

P1 Other than the skateboarding accident, the patient is a normal healthy patient

Units calculation

Units = Base + Time + PS + Emergency = 5+ 7.8 + 0 + 0 = 12.8

Clinical viewpoint

The wound on the left leg required debridement of subcutaneous tissue and skin. Therefore, the correct CPT code was selected. The wound on the right leg was deeper and required debridement of nonviable muscle, subcutaneous tissue, and skin. When coding for debridement, concentrate on how deep the wound penetrates and the square cm.

Case 10: Integumentary system, muscles, and nerves of the head, neck, and posterior trunk

- Anesthesia time: 4:09 P.M. to 4:46 P.M.
- KL, MD Anesthesiologist performed the anesthesia for the case
- Anesthesia: Monitored anesthesia care
- PS II
- A 60-year-old woman presents for a follow-up with a pressure ulcer on her right heel. The wound measures 4 cm x 4 cm. She previously underwent extensive debridement. After review, the physician provides selective active wound care management. The wound was allowed to close by secondary intention. How is this coded?
- Diagnosis: Pressure ulcer of right heel, stage 2
- Procedure: Debridement (e.g. high-pressure waterjet with/without suction, sharp selective debridement with scissors, scalpel, and forceps), open wound (e.g. fibrin, devitalized epidermis and/or dermis, exudate, debris, biofilm), including topical application(s), wound assessment, use of a whirlpool, when performed and instruction(s) for ongoing care, per session, total wound(s) surface area; first 20 sq. cm or less

Codes

L89.612, 97597

ASA Crosswalk Lookup

97597=5 base value units=00300

Overall anesthesiology code for the case

00300-AA-QS-P2

00300 Anesthesia for all procedures on the integumentary system, muscles and nerves of head, neck, and posterior trunk, not otherwise specified

P2 A patient with mild systemic disease; the patient only has one condition; pressure ulcer of heel

Units calculation = Base + Time + PS + Emergency = 5 + 2.47 + 0 + 0 = 7.4

If the patient were a Medicare patient,

Medicare units = Base + Time = 5 + 2.47 = 7.4

Clinical viewpoint

Selective active care wound management involves debridement of the epidermis and dermis only, and therefore the code is 97597.

Case 11: Lumbar region

- Anesthesia time: 06:00 A.M. to 10:00 A.M.
- PW, MD Anesthesiologist performed the anesthesiology for the case while directing five concurrent cases
- Anesthesia: General endotracheal
- Anesthesiologist placed a radial arterial catheter and Swan Ganz catheter at beginning of the case.
- PS I
- A 50-year-old female presents with debilitating back pain with radiation to the right leg and numbness and tingling for two years. She was otherwise healthy.
- MRI scan shows thecal sac compression at L5-S1 facet joint and nerve root compression at L5-S1.
- Diagnosis: Thecal sac compression L5-S1; nerve root compression L5-S1
- Procedure: Laminectomy, facetectomy, and foraminotomy L5-S1 for thecal sac decompression and nerve root decompression above and beyond that necessary for the approach to the interspace to perform the interbody fusion; arthrodesis, posterior interbody technique, including laminectomy to prepare interspace (other than for decompression), single interspace; lumbar

Codes

G95.20, G54.8, 22630-RT, 63047-RT

ASA Crosswalk Lookup

63047=8 base value units=00630

22630=8 base value units=00630

In this case, the split tie for the anesthesiology code made no difference. Both anesthesia codes are the same with equal base value units. The first-listed CPT code is 22630-RT (relative value units=45.76) compared to 63047-RT (relative value units 32.06).

Overall anesthesiology code for the case

00630-AD-P1,

36620, 93503

00630 Anesthesia for procedures in lumbar region

AD Medical supervision by a physician; more than four concurrent anesthesia procedures

P1 Physical status modifier Normal healthy patient

Units calculation=Base+Time+PS+Emergency=8+16.0+0=0=24.0

Clinical viewpoint

This is a case outlining both anesthesiology and pain management. Laminectomy involves cutting out of the lamina, part of the neural arch of the vertebra extending from the pedicle to the median line. Facetectomy is cutting out of the facet, or particular part of the intervertebral joint. Foraminotomy means cutting into the foramen, or a narrow passageway on both sides of the vertebra which allow nerve roots to travel from the spinal cord to other parts of the body. Arthrodesis is the surgical fusion of a joint so that the bones grow solidly together. All four of these procedures are necessary to treat the compression of the thecal sac, which surrounds the spinal cord for sheathing and protection, and nerve root compression in this case.

The anesthesiologist performed anesthesiology on more than four concurrent anesthesia procedures and the type of anesthesia was general endotracheal, in which intubation is performed and the patient is not conscious and cannot maintain control over his own airway.

Case 12: Integumentary system, muscles, and nerves of the head, neck, and posterior trunk

- Anesthesia time: 07:00 A.M. to 07:30 A.M.
- FD, MD Anesthesiologist supervised 2 CRNAs for the anesthesiology of the case
- DR, CRNA, WT, CRNA provided anesthesiology for the case under the medical direction of an anesthesiologist
- Anesthesia: General endotracheal
- PS I
- A 17-year-old high school football player accidentally burns his chest on a hot cautery instrument, resulting in a 4 cm X 4 cm burn with blisters. The burn is a second-degree burn.
- Diagnosis: Second-degree burn on chest involving epidermis with penetration into the dermis
- Procedure: Active wound care management of second-degree burn involving debridement of an open wound, epidermis, and dermis, involving topical applications, wound assessment, and instructions for ongoing care

Codes

T21.21XA, T31.0, X16.XXXA, Y93.89, Y92.213, Y99.9, 97597

ASA Crosswalk Lookup

00300=5 base value units=97597

Overall anesthesiology code for the case for the billing anesthesiologist

00300-QK-P1

Overall anesthesiology code for the case for the billing CRNAs

00300-QX-P1

00300 Anesthesia for all procedures on the integumentary system, muscles and nerves of head, neck, and posterior trunk, not otherwise specified

QK Medical direction of two, three, or four concurrent anesthesia procedures involving qualified individuals

QX CRNA service: with medical direction by a physician

P1 A normal healthy patient

Units calculation=7.0

Clinical viewpoint

The football player was burned by a hot instrument and a second-degree burn developed on his chest. The burn involved the integumentary system. A second-degree burn involves penetration into the epidermis and dermis. Active wound care management involves a debridement of the dermis and epidermis only, not the subcutaneous tissue. The burn was 16 sq. cm. The anesthesia was for the debridement of the integumentary system, or the skin, hair, and nails. The integumentary system has a variety of functions; it may serve to waterproof, cushion, and protect the deeper tissues, which for this case is important for protecting the deeper tissues against the threat of a burn.

Case 13: Integumentary system on the extremities, anterior trunk, and perineum

- Anesthesia time 08:00 A.M. to 10:49 A.M.
- HF, MD Anesthesiologist performed the anesthesiology for the case while directing one CRNA
- KF, CRNA was the CRNA for the case
- KF, CRNA placed a central venous catheter in the subclavian vein
- Anesthesia: General endotracheal
- PS II
- The anesthesiology for the case was complicated by controlled hypotension.
- The pt. is a 35-year-old female with mild gastroesophageal reflux disease. She swims a lot and suffered from cellulitis in both legs. She presents today one week later with extensive cellulitis.
- The provider debrides 25 sq. cm of subcutaneous tissue from the right leg, and 20 sq. cm of subcutaneous tissue from the left leg.
- Calculate units for both Blue Cross Blue Shield of CT and Medicare.
- Diagnosis: Bilateral lower extremity cellulitis; gastroesophageal reflux disease
- Procedures: Debridement of 25 sq. cm of subcutaneous tissue from the right leg; Debridement of 20 sq. cm of subcutaneous tissue from the left leg

Codes

L03.115, L03.116, K21.9, 11042 + 11045 X 2

ASA Crosswalk Lookup

11042=3 base value units=00400

Overall anesthesiology code for the billing anesthesiologist for the case

00400-QY-P2, +99135

Overall anesthesiology code for the CRNA for the case

00400-QX-P2, +99135

36556

00400 Anesthesia for procedures on the integumentary system on the extremities, anterior trunk, and perineum, not otherwise specified

+99135 Anesthesia complicated by utilization of controlled hypotension, corresponding to 5 base value units

Units calculation = Base + Time + PS + Emergency = 3 + 11.2 + 0 + 5 = 19.2 (Can round up or down)

Medicare units = Base + Time= 3 + 11.2 = 14.2 (Can round up or down)

Base units = Base = 3

Time units = Anesthesia time/15 = 169/15 = 11.2

Clinical viewpoint

The code for the central venous catheter, 36556 can also be for the anesthesiologist since he supervised the CRNA for the case. Note that for the debridement, the sq. cm counted for both the right leg and left leg combined; i.e., the debridement codes are additive for the same code (subcutaneous, including dermis and epidermis (in this example). The patient suffered from controlled hypotension during the operation (see units calculation).

For anesthesia modifiers from HCPCS II:

Only two HCPCS II modifiers are correlated for the CRNA: QX, QZ.

For anesthesiologist, the HCPCS II modifiers AA, AD, QK, and QY correlate. These are the only codes for the anesthesiologist.

QS applies to a Monitored anesthesia care (MAC) service

Case 14: Intraoral

- Anesthesia time 09:00 A.M. to 09:59 A.M.
- BN, MD anesthesiologist personally provided the anesthesia for the case
- No CRNAs
- The surgical resident placed the central venous catheter, internal jugular vein
- PS III
- A 15-year-old boy has enlarged tonsils and adenoids. He is examined in detail by his primary care physician and found to have inflammation of the tonsils and adenoids for two years. He undergoes tonsillectomy and adenoidectomy.
- Diagnosis: Chronic tonsillitis and adenoiditis
- Procedure: Tonsillectomy and adenoidectomy

Codes

J35.03, 99214-25, 42821

ASA Crosswalk Lookup

42821=5 base value units=00170

Overall anesthesiology code for the billing anesthesiologist

00170-AA-P3

Units calculation=9.9

Clinical viewpoint

Anesthesia for intraoral procedures, including biopsy; not otherwise specified was provided by the anesthesiologist. The patient is over 12 years old (CPT code 42821). The central venous catheter is not coded for the anesthesiology coding since the surgical resident placed the line. The anesthesiologist, doctor providing the anesthesia, or CRNA must place the central line for the code to be coded for by the billing anesthesiologist. The anesthesiologist personally provided the anesthesia (HCPCS II modifier AA). The patient has severe systemic disease, i.e., chronic tonsillitis and adenoiditis (ICD-10-CM code J35.03).

Case 15: Nose and accessory sinuses

- Anesthesia time: 06:40 A.M. to 11:17 A.M.
- MM, MD Anesthesiologist performed the anesthesia for the case personally
- The anesthesiologist placed a central venous catheter in the internal jugular vein for IV antibiotics
- PS III
- The patient is a 55-year-old female with sinus congestion for two years. He took a course of oral antibiotics for sinusitis two weeks recently. On exam, the forehead is tender with the maxilla. On CT scan and MRI there is inflammation of the frontal sinus and inflammation of the ethmoid sinus.
- Diagnoses: Chronic frontal sinusitis; chronic ethmoidal sinusitis; chronic maxillary sinusitis
- Procedures: Nasal sinus endoscopy, surgical with ethmoidectomy, total (anterior and posterior); Nasal sinus endoscopy, surgical, with maxillary antrostomy; Nasal sinus endoscopy, surgical with frontal sinus exploration with the removal of tissue from the frontal sinus

Codes

J32.1, J32.2, J32.0, 31276-59, 31255, 31256

ASA Crosswalk Lookup

31255=5 base value units=00160

31256=5 base value units=00160

31276=5 base value units=00160

Overall anesthesiology code for the billing anesthesiologist

00160-AA-P3,

36556

Units calculation

Units = Base + Time + PS + Emergency = 5 + 18.4 + 1 + 0 = 24.4 (Can round down or up for CANPC exam)

Clinical viewpoint

The patient has sinusitis on three sinuses as shown by CT and MRI, maxillary, frontal, and ethmoidal. The patient has a severe systemic disease, and therefore a physical status modifier P3. Maxillary antrostomy or opening of an antrum, or cavity of a bone for drainage, total ethmoidectomy, and frontal sinus exploration with the removal of inflamed tissue are performed as treatment of this severe condition. There is a three-way tie from ASA Crosswalk Lookup, but all CPT codes correlate with 00160 for the overall anesthesiology code. The first-listed CPT code is 31276-59 (relative value units=14.44), the second-listed CPT code is 31255 (relative value units=11.45), and the third-listed CPT code is 31256 (relative value units=5.66). The anesthesiologist placed the central venous catheter in the internal jugular vein; therefore, the central venous catheter is coded for in the anesthesiology case.

Case 16: Upper gastrointestinal endoscopic procedures, endoscope introduced proximal to duodenum; endoscopic retrograde cholangiopancreatography (ERCP)

- Anesthesia time 12:00 P.M. to 4:48 P.M.
- Anesthesiologist personally provided the anesthesia for the case
- Anesthesia: General endotracheal
- PS III
- The pt. is a 55-year-old male with a 6-month history of abdominal pain, weight loss, and jaundice. His bilirubin level is elevated. The primary care physician refers the patient to a gastroenterologist, who performs endoscopic retrograde cholangiopancreatography to evaluate the patient for his symptoms and hyperbilirubinemia.
- Diagnosis: Abdominal pain, weight loss, and hyperbilirubinemia
- Procedure: Endoscopic retrograde cholangiopancreatography

Codes

R10.9, R63.4, E80.7, 43260

ASA Crosswalk Lookup

43260=6 base value units=00732

Overall anesthesiology code for billing anesthesiologist

00732-AA-P3

Anesthesia for upper gastrointestinal endoscopic procedures, endoscope introduced proximal to duodenum; endoscopic retrograde cholangiopancreatography (ERCP)

Units calculation=Base+Time+PS+Emergency=6+19.2+1+0=26.2

Clinical viewpoint

This patient required ERCP to evaluate his abdominal pain, weight loss, and hyperbilirubinemia. The patient has the severe systemic disease, correlating with physical status modifier P3. Endoscopic retrograde cholangiopancreatography is an upper gastrointestinal endoscopic procedure in which the endoscope is introduced proximal to the duodenum. The anesthesiologist personally provided the anesthesiology for the case (modifier AA).

Case 17: Male genitalia (including open urethral procedures); vasectomy

- Anesthesia time 10:47 A.M. to 11:36 A.M.
- Anesthesiologist personally provided the anesthesiology for the case
- Anesthesia: General endotracheal
- PS I
- Healthy 55-year-old male with four children has a vasectomy and postoperative semen examination
- Diagnosis: Encounter for sterilization
- Procedure: Bilateral vasectomy including postoperative semen examination

Codes

Z30.2, 55250

ASA Crosswalk Lookup

55250=3 base value units=00921

Overall anesthesiology code for billing anesthesiologist

00921-AA-P1

Units calculation=Base+Time+PS+Emergency=3+3.26+0+0=6.26

00921 Anesthesia for procedures on male genitalia (including open urethral procedures); vasectomy, unilateral or bilateral

AA Anesthesiologist personally provided the anesthesiology for the case

P1 The patient is healthy

Case 18: Open or surgical arthroscopic on knee joint

- Anesthesia time 6:35 P.M. to 10:15 P.M.
- Anesthesiologist personally performs the anesthesia for the case while running five concurrent procedures
- Anesthesia: General endotracheal
- PS I
- A 25-year-old healthy male injures his left knee.
- Diagnosis: Torn medial meniscus, left knee
- Procedures: Arthroscopy with major synovectomy, two or more compartments; Arthroscopy with medial meniscectomy including debridement/shaving of articular cartilage (chondroplasty)

Codes

S83.242A, 29876-LT, 29881-LT

ASA Crosswalk Lookup

29876=4 base value units=01400

29881=4 base value units=01400

Overall anesthesiology code for the billing anesthesiologist

01400-AD-P1

01400 Anesthesia for open or surgical arthroscopic procedures on knee joint; not otherwise specified

AD Medical supervision by a physician; more than four concurrent anesthesia procedures

P1 The patient is a normal healthy patient

Units calculation=18.67

Clinical viewpoint

The patient receives a synovectomy and medial meniscectomy for a torn medial meniscus of the left knee. The anesthesia is for open or surgical arthroscopic procedures on the knee joint. ASA Crosswalk lookup shows a tie, but it makes no difference since the anesthesia code is the same.

Case 19: Eye; lens surgery

- Anesthesia time 8:00 A.M. to 9:01 A.M.
- Anesthesiologist personally provided the anesthesiology for the case
- Anesthesia: General endotracheal
- PS I
- The patient is a 65-year-old female who presents with age-related nuclear cataract of the left eye. He undergoes cataract surgery.
- Diagnosis: Age-related nuclear cataract, left eye
- Procedure: Extracapsular cataract removal with insertion of intraocular lens prosthesis (1-stage procedure), manual or mechanical technique utilizing phacoemulsification

Codes

H25.12, 66984-LT

ASA Crosswalk Lookup

66984=4 base value=00142

Overall anesthesiology code for the billing anesthesiologist

00142-AA, P1

Units calculation=4+4.07+0+0=8.07

Clinical viewpoint

This patient has what is known as an age-related cataract of the nucleus of the lens of the eye. He undergoes cataract surgery utilizing phacoemulsification to remove the cataract and replace the cataract with an intraocular lens prosthesis. The anesthesia was performed for procedures on the eye; lens surgery. The anesthesiologist performed the anesthesiology for the case. The patient is a normal healthy patient.

Case 20: Transurethral (including cystoscopy) procedure; transurethral resection of bladder tumors(s)

- Anesthesia time is 11:06 A.M. to 12:37 A.M.
- Anesthesiologist personally provided the anesthesiology for the case
- Anesthesia: General endotracheal
- PS III
- The patient is a 75-year-old patient with cancer of the anterior wall of the bladder.
- Diagnosis: Malignant neoplasm of the anterior wall of the bladder, 2.5 cm in diameter size
- Procedure: Cystourethroscopy with fulguration (including cryosurgery or laser surgery) and/or resection of MEDIUM bladder tumor(s) (2.0 to 5.0 cm)

Codes

C67.3, 52235

ASA Crosswalk Lookup

52235=5 base value units=00912

Overall anesthesiology code for the billing anesthesiologist

00912-AA-P3,

+99100

Units calculation=Base+Time+PS+Emergency=5+6.07+1+1=13.07

Clinical viewpoint

The patient undergoes cystourethroscopy with resection of a MEDIUM bladder tumor of the anterior wall. The patient has severe systemic disease or cancer (PS III). The patient has a qualifying circumstance, or extreme age greater than seventy.

Case 21: Integumentary system, muscles, and nerves of the head, neck, and posterior trunk

- Anesthesia time is 7:05 A.M. to 8:57 A.M.
- Anesthesiologist provided the anesthesiology for the case
- Anesthesia: General endotracheal
- PS III
- The patient is a 72-year-old male with basal cell carcinoma of the cheek of the face measuring 2.6 cm in diameter and a malignant neoplasm of the right upper arm measuring 3.5 cm in diameter. He presents for excision of both tumors and simple repair.
- Diagnoses: Basal cell carcinoma of the cheek of the face, 2.6 cm; Malignant neoplasm of the right upper limb, 3.5 cm
- Procedures: Excision of basal cell carcinoma of the cheek of the face, excised diameter 2.6 cm; Excision malignant lesion of the upper limb, excised diameter 3.5 cm; Simple repair of superficial wound of extremities, 3.5 cm; simple repair of superficial wound of face, 2.6 cm

Codes

C44.319, C76.41, 11643, 11604, 12002-59, 12013

ASA Crosswalk Lookup

11643=5 base value units=00300

11604=3 base value units=00400

12013=5 base value units=00300

12002=5 base value units=00300

Overall anesthesia code for the billing anesthesiologist

00300-AA-P3,

+99100

00300 Anesthesia for all procedures on the integumentary system, muscles and nerves of the head, neck, and posterior trunk, not otherwise specified

Units calculation=Base+Time+PS+Emergency=5+7.47+1+1=14.47

Clinical viewpoint

The patient has basal cell carcinoma of the face and a malignant neoplasm of the upper limb. The procedures performed were the excision of both malignant tumors and simple repairs. The patient has a severe systemic disease (PS III). There was a three-way tie in anesthesiology coding, yet all three CPT codes yielded the same anesthesia code (00300). The anesthesia code with the highest base unit value is the overall anesthesia code for the case.

Case 22: Integumentary system on the extremities, anterior trunk, and perineum

- Anesthesia time 5:00 P.M. to 6:02 P.M.
- Anesthesiologist provided the anesthesiology for the case
- Anesthesia: General endotracheal
- PS III
- Pt. with a diagnosis of right renal cyst is scheduled to undergo sclerosis of the cyst. Sino gram through the existing drainage tube was performed.
- Diagnosis: Renal cyst, right
- Procedures: Injection of sinus tract; Radiologic examination, sinus tract study; radiological supervision and interpretation

Codes

N28.1, 20500, 76080

ASA Crosswalk Lookup

20500=3 base value units=00400

76080=Not in ASA Crosswalk

Overall anesthesiology code for the billing anesthesiologist

00400-AA, P3

Units calculation=16.4

Clinical viewpoint

The sinus tract study is a radiological examination not requiring anesthesia. The injection of the sinus tract for sclerosis of the renal cyst is coded and determines an anesthesia code. The renal cyst is a severe systemic disease.

Case 23: Anesthesia for intraperitoneal procedures in the upper abdomen including laparoscopy; not otherwise specified

- Anesthesia time 3:24 P.M. to 6:15 P.M.
- Anesthesiologist personally provided the anesthesiology for the case
- Anesthesia: General endotracheal
- PS III
- The pt. has an abdominal hernia causing obstruction and presents for hernia repair.
- Diagnosis: Abdominal ventral hernia causing obstruction; incarcerated
- Procedures: Abdominoplasty; Abdominal wall plication for ventral hernia repair

Codes

K46.0, 15830, 49653

ASA Crosswalk Lookup

15830=5 base value units=00802

49653=7 base value units=00790

Overall anesthesiology code for the case for the billing anesthesiologist

00790-AA-P3

Units calculation=Base+Time+PS+Emergency=7+11.4+1+0=19.4

Clinical viewpoint

The higher base value units for anesthesia code 00790 makes 00790 the overall anesthesiology code for the case

Case 24: Electrophysiological procedures, including radiofrequency ablation

- Anesthesia time 2:05 P.M. to 3:31 P.M.
- Anesthesiologist personally provided the anesthesia for the case
- Anesthesia: General endotracheal
- PS III
- The pt. is a 55-year-old male who presents with ventricular tachycardia. He undergoes ablation with Impella-R support.
- Diagnosis: Ventricular tachycardia
- Procedure: Intracardiac catheter ablation of an arrhythmogenic focus with the treatment of ventricular tachycardia or focus of ventricular ectopy including intracardiac electrophysiological 3D mapping

Codes

I47.2, 93654

ASA Crosswalk Lookup

93654=10 base value units=00537

Overall anesthesiology code for the case for the billing anesthesiologist

00537-AA-P3

Units calculation=Base+Time+PS+Emergency=10+5.73+1+0=16.73

Clinical viewpoint

The patient has ventricular tachycardia requiring intracatheter ablation of an arrhythmogenic focus with the treatment of ventricular tachycardia. The anesthesia for electrophysiological procedures including radiofrequency ablation is performed.

Case 25: Intraperitoneal in the upper abdomen including laparoscopy

- Anesthesia time 7:00 P.M to 9:25 P.M.
- Anesthesiologist personally provided the anesthesiology for the case
- Anesthesia: General endotracheal
- PS III
- Pt. is a 50-year-old female who has severe abdominal pain and undergoes surgery for splenic hemorrhage. Accidental perforation of colonic splenic flexure occurring during surgery.
- Diagnosis: Accidental perforation of colonic splenic flexure during surgery with emergency bleeding
- Procedure: Laparoscopy procedure, spleen

Codes

D73.5, K63.1, 38129

ASA Crosswalk Lookup

38129=unlisted procedure=7 base value units=00790

Overall anesthesiology code for the case for the billing anesthesiologist

00790-AA-P3,

+99140

Units calculation=19.67

Clinical viewpoint

This patient has a splenic hemorrhage and an accidental perforation of colonic splenic flexure as a complication during surgery. Anesthesia for intraperitoneal procedures in the upper abdomen including laparoscopy; not otherwise specified is performed. Anesthesia complicated by emergency conditions (specify) which was the emergency bleeding for the case was performed (+99140) and scored two base value units in the calculation of the unit.

Case 26: Integumentary system, muscles, and nerves of the head, neck, and posterior trunk

- Anesthesia time 9:21 A.M. to 10:37 A.M.
- Anesthesiologist provided general endotracheal anesthesia for the case. A 25-year-old normal healthy patient (P I) has a one-inch by the one-inch second-degree burn on his face. He received an Acellular dermal replacement graft 2.5 cm X 2.5 cm such as Integra for his face.

Codes

T20.20XA, T31.0, 15275, Q4106

ASA Crosswalk Lookup

15275=5 base value units=00300

Overall anesthesiology code for the billing anesthesiologist

00300-AA-P1

Units calculation=10.07

Clinical viewpoint

The patient has a second-degree burn which is less than 10% of the total body surface on his face which requires an Acellular dermal replacement graft such as Integra to replace the dermis. A second-degree burn penetrates into the epidermis and dermis. The anesthesia is for procedures on the integumentary system, muscle, and nerves of head, neck, and posterior trunk, not otherwise specified (00300). In this case, there is one CPT code corresponding to the correct anesthesiology code for the case.

Case 27: Percutaneous image-guided on the spine and spinal cord; therapeutic

- Anesthesia time 4:00 P.M. to 8:14 P.M.
- Anesthesiologist personally performed the general endotracheal anesthesia for the case. The patient is a normal healthy patient who is having a neurostimulator and leads placed percutaneously for chronic back pain, which he has had for two years in an ambulatory surgery care center. During surgery, the placement of the neurostimulator leads was aborted. The spinal neurostimulator pulse generator was placed.

Codes

G89.29, 63650-74, 63685

ASA Crosswalk Lookup

63685=5 base value units=00300

63650=5 base units value=01936

Overall anesthesiology code for the case for the billing anesthesiologist

01936-AA-P1

Units calculation=21.93

Clinical viewpoint

This patient has a discontinued procedure for percutaneous implantation of neurostimulator electrodes, plate/paddle, and epidural (63650-74) for which the neurostimulator pulse generator was placed (63685). The anesthesiology was 01936 Anesthesia for percutaneous image-guided procedures on the spine and spinal cord; therapeutic. In this case, there is a split tie. 63650 is the first-listed code in relative value order with a relative value unit of 11.82 and 63685 is the second-listed code with a relative value unof it 10.54. This case is both anesthesiology and pain management and illustrates the placement of neurostimulator leads for chronic pain from the spinal cord and brain. The neurostimulator is placed under the skin of the abdomen, and the neurostimulator leads give electronic signals to the epidural space near the spinal cord.

Case 28: Partial rib resection

- Anesthesia time 5:00 P.M. to 7:01 P.M.
- Anesthesiologist personally directed the general endotracheal anesthesia for the case. The patient is a normal healthy 27-year-old female who has a VEPTR from a baseball injury five years ago when she had an acquired deformity and presents for adjustment of VEPTR lengthening mechanism. VEPTR stands for Vertical expandable prosthetic titanium rib.

Codes

M95.4, S22.39XS, Z45.89, 21899

ASA Crosswalk Lookup

21899=unlisted code

Overall anesthesia code for the case

00470-AA-P1 Anesthesia for partial rib resection; not otherwise specified

Units calculation=Base+Time+PS+Emergency=6+8.07+0+0=14.07

Clinical viewpoint

When the CPT code looked up in ASA Crosswalk is unlisted, do your best to find an appropriate anesthesiology code based on the descriptions in CPT. The patient presented for an adjustment of VEPTR (Z45.89) which was placed for an acquired deformity of the rib (M95.4) from a baseball injury from five years ago which resulted in a rib fracture (S22.39XS), resulting in the sequela of an acquired deformity now.

Case 29: Upper gastrointestinal endoscopic procedures, endoscope introduced proximal to duodenum; not otherwise specified

- Anesthesia time 9:49 A.M. to 10:29 A.M.
- Anesthesiologist personally provided the general endotracheal anesthesia for the case. The patient is a gastrointestinal disorder patient (PS III) with a percutaneous endoscopic gastrostomy (PEG) tube placed for nutrition. He undergoes esophagogastroduodenoscopy (EGD) and PEG removal.

Codes

K92.9, E46, 43235

ASA Crosswalk Lookup

43235=5 base value units=00731

Overall anesthesiology code for the case for the billing anesthesiologist

00731-AA-P3

Units calculation=8.67

Clinical viewpoint

The patient has a severe systemic disease, i.e., a gastrointestinal disorder (P3) and the anesthesia was for upper gastrointestinal endoscopic procedures.

Case 30: Lumbar region

- Anesthesia time 2:45 P.M. to 5:57 P.M.
- Anesthesiologist personally directed the general endotracheal anesthesia for the case. A normal healthy 35-year-old male patient had back pain for one year. He received an MRI which showed L4-L5 lateral foraminal stenosis and underwent L4-L5 Laminectomy, facetectomy, and foraminotomy with decompression of spinal cord.

Codes

M99.83, 63047

ASA Crosswalk Lookup

63047=8 base value units=00630

Overall anesthesiology code for the case for the billing anesthesiologist

00630-AA-P1

Units calculation=Base+Time+PS+Emergency=8+12.8+0+0=20.8

Clinical viewpoint

The anesthesia is for procedures in the lumbar region. The case is both an anesthesiology and a pain management case. Surgery was required to treat the foraminal stenosis which caused the back pain after medication for pain management was successful only to a degree.

Case 31: Upper abdomen, including laparoscopy

- Anesthesia time 2:14 P.M. to 4:15 P.M.
- Anesthesiologist provided the general endotracheal anesthesia for the case. A normal healthy patient (PS I) complains of right upper quadrant pain. A CT scan shows acute cholecystitis. A laparoscopic surgical cholecystectomy is performed.

Codes

K81.0, 47562

ASA Crosswalk Lookup

47562=7 base value units=00790

Overall anesthesiology code for the case for the billing anesthesiologist

00790-AA-P1

Units calculation=15.07

Clinical viewpoint

The patient underwent laparoscopic surgical cholecystectomy under Anesthesia for procedures in upper abdomen including laparoscopy (00790).

Case 32: Intraperitoneal procedure in the upper abdomen

- Anesthesia time from 12:00 P.M. to 3:05 P.M.
- Anesthesiologist provided the general endotracheal anesthesia for the case. A normal healthy patient (PS I) complains of right upper quadrant pain for two years. A CT scan shows chronic cholecystitis. An open cholecystectomy is performed.

Codes

K81.1, 47600

ASA Crosswalk Lookup

47600=7 base value units=00790

Overall anesthesiology code for the billing anesthesiologist

00790-AA-P1

Units calculation=19.33

Clinical viewpoint

The anesthesia is for intraperitoneal procedures in upper abdomen. The procedure was an open procedure. The gall bladder is located in the right upper quadrant.

Case 33: Esophagus

- Anesthesia time 1:58 P.M. to 3:50 P.M.
- Anesthesiologist personally directed the general endotracheal anesthesia for the case. A 50-year-old male patient has had difficulty swallowing and gastroesophageal reflux disease for two years (PS III). He is found on MRI to have weakness of the lower esophageal sphincter. He undergoes laparoscopic augmentation of the lower esophageal sphincter with a magnetic device (e.g., LINX Reflux Management System).

Codes

K21.9, M62.89, 43289

ASA Crosswalk Lookup

43289=unlisted code=7 base value units=00500

Overall anesthesiology code for the case for the billing anesthesiologist

00500-AA-P3

Units calculation=23.47

Clinical viewpoint

The anesthesia was for procedures on the esophagus. In this case, the CPT code was for an unlisted procedure and therefore not listed in ASA Crosswalk. In this case, it is important to select a code from the CPT book.

Case 34: Therapeutic interventional radiological procedure involving the arterial system; carotid or coronary

- Anesthesia time is 7:05 P.M. to 9:38 P.M.
- Anesthesiologist provided the general endotracheal anesthesia for the case. The patient is a 50-year-old female with atherosclerosis (PS III) of her left anterior descending coronary artery on an angiogram. Percutaneous transluminal angioplasty, atherectomy, and stent insertion were performed on the left anterior descending coronary artery.

Codes

I25.10, 92933-LD

ASA Crosswalk Lookup

92933=8 base value units=01925

Units calculation=19.2

Overall anesthesiology code for the case

01925-AA-P3

Clinical viewpoint

The patient has three cardiovascular procedures performed on the same branch (LAD) of the left coronary artery, percutaneous transluminal angioplasty, atherectomy, and stent insertion. One CPT code (92933-LD) accounts for all three procedures performed on the same vessel. Anesthesia for therapeutic interventional radiological procedures involving the arterial system; carotid or coronary is performed (01925).

Case 35: Open on bones of the lower leg, ankle, and foot; osteotomy or osteoplasty

- Anesthesia time 4:48 P.M. to 9:45 P.M.
- Anesthesiologist personally directed the monitored anesthesia care for the case. The patient is a 45-year-old male with osteoarthritis (PS III) who sustained a displaced bimalleolar right ankle fracture from an automobile accident two years ago. He underwent open treatment for the fracture involving the placement of hardware. Today, he presents with right ankle pain from osteoarthritis. He undergoes arthrodesis of the ankle (ankle fusion), osteotomy, and removal of hardware.

Codes

M19.071, S82.841S, V89.2XXS, 27870, 27705, 27704

ASA Crosswalk Lookup

27870=3 base value units=01480

27705=4 base value units=01484

27704=3 base value units=01480

Overall anesthesiology code for the billing anesthesiologist

01484-AA-QS-P3

Units calculation=Base+Time+PS+Emergency=4+19.8+1+0=24.8

Clinical viewpoint

The patient underwent open arthrodesis of the ankle (27870), osteotomy of the tibia (27705), and removal of ankle implant (hardware) (27704) for ankle pain secondary to osteoarthritis. The patient has sequelae from the displaced bimalleolar ankle fracture (S82.841S) sustained from an automobile accident (V89.2XXS) two years ago. In ASA Crosswalk Lookup, because 01484 is 4 base value units, higher than the other two codes, the overall anesthesiology for the case is 01484. The anesthesia is for open procedures on bones of the lower leg, ankle, and foot; osteotomy or osteoplasty of tibia and/or fibula.

Case 36: Intracranial

- Anesthesia time 4:00 A.M. to 8:04 A.M.
- Anesthesiologist provided the general endotracheal anesthesia for the case. A 25-year-old male patient has epilepsy (PS IV), not intractable without status epilepticus. He undergoes amygdalohippocampectomy by stereotactic method for subcortical structures.

Codes

G40.909, 61566

ASA Crosswalk Lookup

61566=11 base value units=00210

Overall anesthesiology code for the case for the billing anesthesiologist

00210-AA-P4

Units calculation=Base+Time+PS+Emergency=11+16.27+2+0=29.27

Clinical viewpoint

The patient undergoes Craniotomy with an elevation of bone flap for selective amygdalohippocampectomy (61566) for epilepsy (G40.909), a severe systemic disease that is a constant threat to life (PS IV). Anesthesia is for intracranial procedures, not otherwise specified (00210).

Case 37: Heart, pericardial sac, and great vessels of the chest; with pump

- Anesthesia time 9:24 P.M. to 12:15 A.M.
- Anesthesiologist provided the general endotracheal anesthesia including cardiopulmonary bypass (PS III) for the case. A 38-year-old female complains of palpitations. On physical exam, the doctor finds a heart murmur. Transthoracic echocardiogram with image documentation (2D) including M-mode recording, complete shows mitral valve stenosis. The patient undergoes valvuloplasty, mitral valve, with cardiopulmonary bypass, with Carpentier prosthetic ring.

Codes

I34.2, 33426, 93307

ASA Crosswalk Lookup

33426=20 base value units=00562

Overall anesthesiology code for the case for the billing anesthesiologist

00562-AA-P3

Units calculation=32.4

Clinical viewpoint

The patient has a heart murmur secondary to mitral valve stenosis (I34.2) according to an echocardiogram. The patient undergoes valvuloplasty of the mitral valve with a cardiopulmonary bypass with a prosthetic ring (33426). The anesthesia is for procedures on the heart, pericardial sac, and great vessels of the chest; with a pump (00562). The case was an intense case as it required cardiopulmonary bypass and therefore general endotracheal anesthesia was required.

Case 38: Thoracic spine and cord, via an anterior transthoracic approach; utilizing 1 lung ventilation

- Anesthesia time 2:05 A.M. to 6:55 A.M.
- Anesthesiologist personally provided the general endotracheal anesthesia for the case (PS III). A 75-year-old female patient with generalized osteoarthritis has had neck and back pain for two years. MRI of the spinal canal and contents, cervical and thoracic, without contrast reveals cervicothoracic disc displacement. The patient undergoes anterior C7-T1 cervical thoracic fusion with total discectomy.

Codes

M50.23, M19.90, 22556, 22222, 72146, 72141

ASA Crosswalk Lookup

22556=15 base value units=00626

22222=15 base value units=00626

Overall anesthesiology code for the billing anesthesiologist

00626-AA-P3,

+99100

Units calculation=36.33

Clinical viewpoint

The patient has cervical disc displacement (M50.23) requiring arthrodesis with anterior interbody technique including minimal discectomy to prepare interspace (22556) and osteotomy of the spine including discectomy (22222). In this case, there is a split tie in anesthesiology coding but it makes no difference since the generated anesthesiology code (00626) is the same for both procedure codes. 22556 is the first-listed code in relative value order.

Case 39: Intraperitoneal in the lower abdomen including laparoscopy

- Anesthesia time 4:15 P.M to 6:02 P.M.
- Anesthesiologist provided the monitored anesthesia care (MAC) for the case (PS I). A 27-year-old healthy female in the second trimester (25th week) of pregnancy presents for maternal care to the OB-GYN doctor. The OB-GYN doctor finds a retro version of the gravid uterus on physical exam and ultrasound. The patient undergoes surgery for anteversion of the retroverted uterus.

Codes

O34.532, Z3A.25, 58540

ASA Crosswalk Lookup

58540=6 base units value=00840

Overall anesthesiology code for the case for the billing anesthesiologist

00840-AA-QS-P1

Units calculation=Base+Time+PS+Emergency=15+19.33+0+0=34.33

Clinical viewpoint

The anesthesia is for intraperitoneal procedures in the lower abdomen including laparoscopy; not otherwise specified (00840). The OB-GYN case involved intraperitoneal surgery on the lower abdomen. The surgery was hysteroplasty, a repair of uterine anomaly.

Case 40: Second- and third-degree burn excision or debridement, with or without skin grafting, at any site, for total body surface area (TBSA) treated during anesthesia or surgery

- Anesthesia time 2:25 P.M. to 3:57 P.M.
- Anesthesiologist personally provided the general endotracheal anesthesia for the case. A healthy 25-year-old patient (P1) becomes burned in the chest wall while removing hot food from the oven. The second-degree partial thickness burn covers approximately 3.5% of the total body surface area. The burn is debrided in the operating room with a dressing placed post-operatively.

Codes

T21.21XA, T31.0, X10.1XXA, Y93.G3, Y92.010, Y99.8, 16020

ASA Crosswalk Lookup

16020=3 base value units=01951

Overall anesthesiology code for the billing anesthesiologist

01951-AA-P1

Units calculation=9.13

Clinical viewpoint

The patient has a second-degree burn extending partial thickness into the dermis which is debrided in the operating room with a dressing placed post-operatively. The anesthesia is for second and third-degree burn excision or debridement with or without skin grafting, any site, for total body surface area (TBSA) treated during anesthesia and surgery; less than 4% total body surface area (01951).

Case 41: Heart, pericardial sac, and great vessels of the chest; with pump oxygenator, age 1 or older, for non-coronary bypass procedures (eg. valve procedures) or for re-operation for coronary bypass more than 1 month after the original operation

- Anesthesia time 4:45 P.M. to 8:17 P.M.
- Anesthesiologist personally provided the general endotracheal anesthesia for the case (PS III). A 1.5-year-old female has a congenital malformation of the aorta. She has a murmur on the cardiac exam and is found to have aortic valve insufficiency, non-rheumatic on transthoracic echocardiogram. The patient undergoes aortic root replacement with thoracic aorta replacement with cardiopulmonary bypass.

Codes

Q25.40, I35.1, 33863

ASA Crosswalk Lookup

33863=20 base unit value=00562

Overall anesthesiology code for the case for the billing anesthesiologist

00562-AA-P3

Units calculation=35.1

Clinical viewpoint

The anesthesia is for procedures on heart, pericardial sac, and great vessels of chest; with pump oxygenator, greater than 1 year of age (00562). The patient has a congenital malformation of the aorta requiring surgery (33863).

Case 42: Heart, pericardial sac, and great vessels of the chest with pump oxygenator, age 1 year or older, for all non-coronary bypass procedures

- Anesthesia time 2:02 P.M. to 6:00 P.M.
- Anesthesiologist personally provided the general endotracheal anesthesia for the case (PS III). The patient is a 56-year-old male with multiple medical problems: atherosclerosis of the aorta, chronic constrictive pericarditis, and an acquired cardiac septal defect. The patient undergoes aortic valve surgery with the excision of calcium deposits. He undergoes resection or incision of subvalvular tissue for discrete subvalvular aortic stenosis.

Codes

I70.0, I31.1, I51.0, 33415

ASA Crosswalk Lookup

33415=20 base value units=00562

Overall anesthesiology code for the case for the billing anesthesiologist

00562-AA-P3

Units calculation=36.87

Clinical viewpoint

The patient has severe medical problems (P3) requiring aortic valve surgery with the excision of calcium deposits. Anesthesia (00562) is for procedures on the heart, pericardial sac, and great vessels of the chest with a pump oxygenator, age 1 year or older, for all non-coronary bypass procedures.

Case 43: Direct coronary artery bypass grafting; with pump oxygenator

- Anesthesia time 4:00 P.M. to 8:25 P.M.
- Anesthesiologist personally provided the general endotracheal anesthesia for the case (PS III). A 55-year-old female patient has atherosclerotic heart multi-vessel disease of the native coronary artery with unstable angina pectoris. She has had cardiac chest pain for over two years. A coronary angiogram performed one week ago showed 90% stenosis in the left anterior descending artery (LAD), 85% stenosis in the right posterior descending artery, 85% stenosis in the obtuse marginal artery (OM) of the left circumflex, and 85% in the Diagonal artery of the left coronary artery. She undergoes an aortocoronary bypass graft utilizing Y-graft and was placed on cardiopulmonary bypass. She undergoes cardiopulmonary bypass utilizing the arterial graft left inferior mesenteric artery (LIMA) graft to the LAD; 3 venous grafts, saphenous vein graft to the right posterior descending artery, saphenous vein graft to the obtuse marginal (OM), and saphenous vein graft to the Diagonal.

Codes

I25.110, 33533+33519

ASA Crosswalk Lookup

33533=18 base value units=00567

33519=not a primary procedure code

Overall anesthesiology code for the case for the billing anesthesiologist

00567-AA-P3

Units calculation=36.67

Clinical viewpoint

The cardiac patient has severe (PS III) multi-vessel coronary artery disease and undergoes an aortocoronary bypass graft utilizing Y-graft. She was placed on cardiopulmonary bypass requiring a 4-vessel coronary artery bypass graft (CABG), three venous for combined arterial-venous grafting, and one arterial (33533+33519). The anesthesia (00567) is for direct coronary artery bypass grafting; with a pump oxygenator.

Case 44: Non-invasive imaging

Anesthesia time is 6:00 P.M. to 7:01 P.M.

The anesthesiologist personally provided the monitored anesthesia care (MAC) for the case (PS III). A 55-year-old male with a history of coronary artery disease presents with chest pains. He undergoes Myocardial perfusion imaging tomographic (SPECT), and multiple studies with stress exercise. SPECT scan finds myocardial ischemia.

Codes

I25.10, I25.5, 78452

ASA Crosswalk Lookup

78452=not listed

01922 as listed in CPT book Anesthesia for non-invasive imaging or radiation therapy

Overall anesthesiology code for the case for the billing anesthesiologist

01922-AA-QS-P3

Units calculation=12.07

Clinical viewpoint

The patient presented with chest pain and was found to have myocardial ischemia on SPECT Myocardial perfusion tomographic imaging (78452). The CPT code 78452 is not listed in ASA Crosswalk. The corresponding anesthesia code is for anesthesia for non-invasive imaging (01922). The anesthesia is monitored anesthesia care (MAC) (QS).

Case 45: Vaginal procedure (including biopsy of labia, vagina, cervix, or endometrium); vaginal hysterectomy

- Anesthesia time is 12:02 P.M. to 3:27 P.M.
- Anesthesiologist personally provided the general endotracheal anesthesia for the case (PS III). A 57-year-old female patient has a benign tumor of the vagina with a tubo-ovarian abscess not responsive to antibiotics from one week ago. The patient undergoes an open vaginal hysterectomy for a 250-g uterus and a bilateral salpingo-oophorectomy. The surgery had emergency bleeding.

Codes

D28.1, N70.03, N99.61, 58262

ASA Crosswalk Lookup

58262=6 base value units=00944

Overall anesthesiology code for the case for the billing anesthesiologist

00944-AA-P3,

+99140

Units calculation=Base+Time+PS+Emergency=6+13.67+1+2=22.67

Clinical viewpoint

Look up the neoplasm code (D28.1) in the neoplasm table. The anesthesia (00944) is for vaginal procedures (including biopsy of labia, vagina, cervix, or endometrium); vaginal hysterectomy. In this case, there was an Emergency or qualifying circumstance of anesthesia complicated by emergency conditions (+99140), i.e. emergency bleeding which is worth 2 base value units in the units calculation in Relative value guide.

Case 46: Open or surgical arthroscopy on the humeral head and neck, sternoclavicular joint, acromioclavicular joint, and shoulder joint

Anesthesia time 2:05 P.M. to 4:07 P.M.

- Anesthesiologist provided the general endotracheal anesthesia for the case. The patient is a healthy 25-year-old male (PS I) who pulled his left shoulder while playing baseball. On physical exam, he is found by his physician to have a left rotator cuff tear secondary to trauma. He underwent arthroscopic rotator cuff repair.

Codes

S46.012A, X58.XXXA, Y93.64, Y92.320, Y99.8, 29827

ASA Crosswalk Lookup

29827=5 base value=01630

Overall anesthesiology code for the billing anesthesiologist

01630-AA-P1

Units calculation=21.13

Clinical viewpoint

The anesthesia (01630) is for open or surgical arthroscopic procedures on the humeral head and neck, sternoclavicular joint, acromioclavicular joint, and shoulder joint; not otherwise specified. The patient has a rotator cuff tear involving a strain of muscles and tendons (S46.012A) secondary to trauma from playing baseball.

Case 47: Open or surgical arthroscopy on the humeral head and neck, sternoclavicular joint, acromioclavicular joint, and shoulder joint; not otherwise specified

- Anesthesia time 4:47 P.M. to 6:39 P.M.
- Anesthesiologist provided general endotracheal anesthesia. The patient is a healthy 30-year-old female (PS I) who suffers from impingement symptoms of the left shoulder dating back to a motorcycle accident. She was seen for a diagnostic left shoulder arthroscopy with arthroscopic subacromial decompression and debridement.

Codes

M75.42, V29.9XXS, 29822, +29826

ASA Crosswalk Lookup

29822=5 base value units=01630

29826=NOT A PRIMARY PROCEDURE CODE

Overall anesthesiology code for the case for the billing anesthesiologist

01630-AA-P1

Units calculation=12.47

Clinical viewpoint

The patient suffers from impingement syndrome of the left shoulder (M75.42) from a motorcycle accident (V29.9XXS). The base value units=5 for 01630. Anesthesia is for open or surgical arthroscopic procedures on the humeral head and neck, sternoclavicular joint, acromioclavicular joint, and shoulder joint.

Case 48: Percutaneous image-guided on the spine and spinal cord; therapeutic

- Anesthesia time 1:17 P.M. to 4:49 P.M.
- Anesthesiologist provided the general endotracheal anesthesia for the case (PS I). The patient is a 25-year-old healthy male (PS I) who fell during a skiing accident two months ago. He was found to have an intervertebral disc displacement (L5-S1) with myelopathy. He underwent a percutaneous laminotomy with transforaminal endoscopic discectomy with ultra-minimally invasive microdiscectomy and foraminotomy.

Codes

M51.06, V00.321D, Y93.23, Y92.838, Y99.8, 0275T

ASA Crosswalk Lookup

0275T=5 base value units=01936

Overall anesthesiology code for the case

01936-AA-P1

Total units calculation for a 3.5-hour operation

Total Units = Base + Time + PS + Emergency = Total units = 5+14.13+0+0=19.13

Clinical viewpoint

The patient received anesthesia for percutaneous image-guided procedures on the spine and spinal cord; therapeutic (01936). The procedure code (0275T) is a T code.

Case 49: Integumentary system on the extremities, anterior trunk, and perineum; radical or modified radical procedure on the breast

- Anesthesia time 2:55 P.M. to 8:59 P.M.
- Anesthesiologist provided the general endotracheal anesthesia for the case (PS IV), supervising two CRNAs. The anesthesiologist placed a left internal jugular central venous catheter and a right radial arterial line prior to the beginning of the case. A 45-year-old female patient with multifocal breast cancer presents to have a total right-modified radical mastectomy with sentinel lymph node injection and biopsy. Subcutaneous tissue was dissected down and flaps were elevated to the clavicle, sternum, and rectus fascia. The breast was pulled medially and dissected out of the right axilla area. Two blue-stained sentinel nodes were removed and additional enlarged nodes were removed and sent for frozen section.

Codes

C50.911, 19307, 38792, 88307, 88331+88332 x 7

ASA Crosswalk Lookup

19307=5 base value units=00404

38792=anesthesia care not typically required

Overall anesthesiology code for the case for the billing anesthesiologist

00404-QK-P4,

36556, 36620

Overall anesthesiology code for the case for the billing CRNA

00404-QX-P4

Total units for a 6-hour operation

Total units = Base + Time + PS + Emergency = 5+24.26+2+0=31.26

Clinical viewpoint

The breast cancer patient (C50.911) underwent modified radical mastectomy (19307) involving surgical removal of the breast, dissection into the axilla, staining of two sentinel nodes (38792), and removal of the two sentinel lymph nodes. The anesthesia (00404) is for procedures on the integumentary system on the extremities, anterior trunk, and perineum; radical or modified radical procedures on the breast. PS IV yields 2 units on the units calculation. The anesthesiologist directs 2 CRNAs (QK). CRNA service is with medical direction by a physician (QX).

Case 50: External, middle, and inner ear including biopsy

- Anesthesia time: 8:00 A.M. to 12:02 P.M.
- Anesthesiologist performed the general endotracheal anesthesia for the case (PS III). A 35-year-old male patient is suffering from chronic mastoiditis, hearing loss, and tympanic membrane perforation. He has sustained facial palsy from one of the prior surgeries and now presents for radical mastoidectomy, facial nerve decompression, and debridement, mastoid obliteration, and a temporalis muscle flap rotation.

Codes

H70.10, H72.90, G51.0, 69603, 15733

ASA Crosswalk Lookup

69603=5 base value units=00120

15733=5 base value units=00300

Overall anesthesiology code for the billing anesthesiologist

00120-AA-P3

Units calculation=22.13

Clinical viewpoint

The overall anesthesiology code is 00120 Anesthesia for procedures on the external, middle, and inner ear including biopsy; is not otherwise specified. In this case, there was a tie in ASA Crosswalk Lookup. The first listed CPT code with the corresponding anesthesiology code breaks the tie. In this case, a revision mastoidectomy; resulting in radical mastoidectomy is listed as the first CPT code (69603).

Case 51: Intraperitoneal procedure in the lower abdomen, including laparoscopy

- Postoperative diagnosis: Acute suppurative appendicitis
- Procedure: Laparoscopic appendectomy
- Anesthesia: General endotracheal and local
- Anesthesiologist performed the general endotracheal anesthesia for the case overseeing 2 CRNAs (PS III).
- Anesthesia time: 2 hours
- Blood loss: Minimal to none
- Complications: None
- Description of procedure: The 45-year-old male patient was brought into the OR. General anesthesia was induced without difficulty. Opt iView technique was used to enter the abdominal cavity via the supraumbilical midline. Inspection of the abdominal cavity showed an inflammatory process in the right lower quadrant, easily identifying the appendix as the source. The appendix was transected at the base of the cecum without difficulty. The appendix was placed in an Endocatch and removed via the 12-mm trocar site. I then irrigated 2 liters of normal saline in the abdominal cavity. I aspirated over the dome of the liver, the right lower quadrant, and pelvis. No surrounding injury to any bowel. No other interloop abscess is identified. The patient tolerated the procedure well. I released the pneumoperitoneum and injected all trocar sites with Marcaine, closed the skin with 4-0 Monocryl and Dermabond.

Codes

44970, K35.80

ASA Crosswalk Lookup

44970=6 base value units=00840

Overall anesthesiology code for the billing anesthesiologist

00840-QK-P3

Overall anesthesiology code for the billing CRNA

00840-QX-P3

Total Units calculation = Base + Time + PS + Emergency = 6+8.0+1+0=14.0

Clinical viewpoint

The patient has acute suppurative appendicitis (PS III) requiring laparoscopic appendectomy. The anesthesia (00840) was for intraperitoneal procedures in the lower abdomen including laparoscopy; not otherwise specified. In this case, the anesthesiologist (QK) directed 2 CRNAs (QX) for the anesthesiology case.

Case 52: Integumentary system on the extremities, anterior trunk, and perineum

- Indications: The patient is a 62-year-old female who presented to Dr. Optum's office with an abnormal mammogram of the right breast. The film a suspicious area on the right breast with microcalcifications and a nonpalpable mass. After a discussion with the patient about the best options on how to proceed, it was decided to perform a needle-localized breast biopsy.
- Postoperative diagnosis: Right breast mass
- Procedure: Needle-localized excisional biopsy of the right breast
- Anesthesia: General endotracheal
- Anesthesiologist personally performed the general endotracheal anesthesia for the case (PS III).
- Anesthesia time: 3.50 hours
- Description of procedure: The patient was brought to the procedure room. The needle had been previously placed in the lesion in the right breast by radiology. After IV sedation was given, the patient was then prepped and draped in the normal sterile fashion.
- After anesthetizing the skin with 0.25% Marcaine and 1% lidocaine mixture, an incision was made with a #10 blade scalpel. The lesion with a needle was then grasped with an Allis clamp. Using a #10 blade scalpel, the specimen was colonized out and sent to radiology for confirmation. Next, hemostasis was obtained using electrobovie cautery. The skin was then closed with #4-0 Monocryl suture in a subcuticular fashion. Steri-Strips and a sterile dressing were applied to the surgical wound. The patient tolerated the procedure quite well and left the procedure well and left the procedure room in stable condition.
- Intraoperative findings
- Nonpalpable right breast mass, excised and sent to radiology with confirmation that the mass is in the specimen.

Codes

19083-RT, 88307, N63.10, R92.0

ASA Crosswalk Lookup

19083=3 base value units=00400

Overall anesthesiology code for the billing anesthesiologist

00400-AA-P3

Units calculation = Base + time + PS + Emergency = 3+14.0+1+0=17.0

Clinical viewpoint

The patient had microcalcifications on a mammogram (R92.0) which was found to be a breast mass in the OR (N63). She has a specimen that was removed from the right breast with a needle-localized excisional biopsy (19037) and sent to pathology (88307). The anesthesia (00400) was for procedures on the integumentary system on the extremities, anterior trunk, and perineum; not otherwise specified. In this case, it is important to remember that the breast is part of the integumentary system.

Case 53: Esophagus, thyroid, larynx, trachea, and lymphatic system of the neck; age 1 year and older

- Postoperative diagnosis: Bilateral cervical lymphadenopathy
- Procedure: Biopsy of right posterior triangle cervical node
- Anesthesia: General endotracheal; Xylocaine 1% with epinephrine supplemented with IV sedation
- Anesthesiology was performed by an anesthesiologist directing one CRNA (PS III)
- Anesthesia time: 1.05 hours
- Findings: A 10 x 8 mm node was present in the posterior triangle of the right neck. This was readily palpable, removed, and sent fresh for flow cytometry and histology.
- Estimated blood loss: Minimal
- Description of procedure: The patient is a 71-year-old male. Under satisfactory preoperative medicine, the patient was taken to the operating room. The right neck was prepped with Chloraprep and draped in the usual sterile manner. The palpable node was marked with a marking pen. The skin, subcutaneous tissue, and subplatysmal tissue were infiltrated with 1% Xylocaine with epinephrine. A transverse incision was made, and the platysma muscle was split in the direction of its fibers. The lymph node was identified and very carefully dissected from the surrounding tissue. No bleeding was encountered. The node was sent fresh. The platysma was closed with a running simple suture of 4-0 Vicryl. The skin was closed with a running subcuticular suture of 4-0 Vicryl.

Codes

38520-RT, 88305, 88182+88314, R59.1

ASA Crosswalk Lookup

38520=6 base value units=00320

Overall anesthesiology code for the billing anesthesiologist

00320-QY-P3, +99100

Overall anesthesiology code for the billing CRNA

00320-QX-P3, +99100

Units calculation: Base+Time+PS+Emergency=

6+4.2+1+1=12.2

Clinical viewpoint

The case is bilateral cervical lymphadenopathy (R59.1) with a biopsy of the right posterior triangle open deep cervical lymph node, generalized as it was bilateral (38520). The anesthesia (00320) is for all procedures on the esophagus, thyroid, larynx, and lymphatic system of the neck; not otherwise specified, age 1 year or older. The specimen was removed and sent to pathology for flow cytometry (88182) and histology (+88314).

Case 54: Integumentary system, muscles, and nerves of the head, neck, and posterior trunk

- Postoperative diagnosis: Large primary basal cell carcinoma of the skin of the left hip
- Procedures: Wide excision of basal cell carcinoma of the left hip
- Intermediate layered closure with extensive mobilization of skin flaps
- Jackson-Pratt drain into the wound
- Anesthesia: General endotracheal; IV sedation by the anesthesiology department and 30 mL of 0.25% Marcaine plain locally
- Anesthesiologist personally provided the general endotracheal anesthesia for the case while directing 5 procedures concurrently (PS IV)
- Anesthesia time: 50 minutes
- Complications: None
- Estimated blood loss: Minimal
- Specimens Removed: A 15 cc X 6.5 cm X 3 cm area of skin and subcutaneous tissues of the left hip containing the patient's large irregular basal cell carcinoma
- Procedure Description: The patient was taken to the operating room. She was given IV sedation by the anesthesiology department. Cancer itself measured 6.6 cm X 5.2 cm in size. Using a marking pen, I then marked off an obliquely oriented elliptical incision measuring 15 cm in length X 6.5 cm in width at its widest point. I then infiltrated the incision line with 30 mL of 0.25% Marcaine without epinephrine.
- Using a #10 blade scalpel, an incision was made and carried all the way down to the muscular fascia circumferentially. Then, using a Bovie electrocautery unit, the skin, and subcutaneous tissues, as well as cancer, were then divided off of the fascia. The specimen was marked with sutures for proper orientation. Once this was done, I extensively undermined the entire wound circumferentially for a distance of at least 5 cm in all directions. Once having done this, the wound would come together with mild tension. A 10 mm Jackson-Pratt drain was placed at the base of the wound and brought out through a separate stab wound inferiorly. It was secured with a 2-0 silk suture. The wound was copiously irrigated out with saline containing bacitracin. The wound was then closed in three layers with interrupted sutures of 2-0 Vicryl for the deep subcutaneous tissues and a running 3-0 Vicryl for the superficial subcutaneous tissues. The skin was closed with interrupted vertical mattress sutures of 4-0 nylon. The drain was then connected to suction. A large bulky dressing was applied. The patient was then moved to the recovery room in stable condition.

Codes

27043, 12032, 88305, C44.719

Overall anesthesiology code for the billing anesthesiologist

00300-AD-P4

Units calculation= 10.33

Clinical viewpoint

The patient has basal cell carcinoma of the skin of the left hip (C44.719) size 6.6 cm X 5.2 cm. Note that the basal cell carcinoma was of the skin as seen in the operative report. The patient underwent excision, tumor, the soft tissue of pelvis and hip area, subcutaneous, 3 cm or greater (27043) and repair, intermediate, wounds of scalp, axillae, trunk and/or extremities (excluding hands and feet; 2.6 cm X 7.5 cm (12032). Note that Intermediate layered closure with extensive mobilization of skin flaps was performed and coded separately in this case. The specimen 15 cc X 6.5 cm X 3 cm of skin and subcutaneous tissues was sent to pathology (88305).

Case 55: Hernia repairs in the lower abdomen; not otherwise specified

- Postoperative diagnosis: Left inguinal hernia
- Cord lipoma
- Procedure performed: Left inguinal hernia repair with mesh
- Findings: Indirect inguinal hernia noted
- Specimens received: Cord lipoma
- Hernia sac
- Left ilioinguinal nerve
- Surgeon: Dr. Optum
- Estimated blood loss: Minimal
- Anesthesia: General endotracheal plus 10 ml of 0.25% Marcaine
- Anesthesiologist provided the anesthesia for the case directing 2 CRNAs (PS II)
- Anesthesia time: 1.05 hours
- Complications: None
- Indications for Procedure: The patient is a pleasant 76-year-old gentleman who presents with a large reducible left inguinal hernia. Risks, benefits, and complications were explained to him in great detail and he wished to proceed.
- Procedure: The patient was taken to the operating room. General anesthesia was administered without incident. We proceeded to use 0.25% Marcaine to anesthetize the area in a field block fashion. We then used a 4-cm incision in the left inguinal crease just below the inguinal ligament and dissected around the skin and subcutaneous tissue and through the Scarpa's fascia down to the external oblique fascia. The external oblique was opened to the external inguinal ring. The ilioinguinal nerve was preserved. We then cut around the spermatic cord at the pubic tubercle with a Penrose drain. We then dissected the anteromedial indirect inguinal hernia sac away from the spermatic cord. There was also a large cord lipoma, and this was resected. We then did a high ligation of the hernia sac with a 2-0 Vicryl suture in a running fashion. We placed it back into the internal inguinal ring. We then closed the internal inguinal ring with a 0 PDS in a figure-of-eight interrupted fashion.
- We then placed out the mesh. We then created a new internal inguinal ring using the same Prolene suture and making it a snug, not a tight, fit.

Codes

49505, 55520-59, +49568, 88304, 88302, K40.90, D17.6

Overall anesthesiology code for the billing anesthesiologist

00830-QK-P2,

+99100

Overall anesthesiology code for the billing CRNA

00830-QX-P2,

+99100

Units calculation=9.2

Clinical viewpoint

The postoperative diagnosis is coded. This is a patient with a unilateral inguinal hernia without obstruction or gangrene (K40.90) and a spermatic cord lipoma (D17.6) who presents for left inguinal hernia repair, reducible with mesh (49505+49568) who in addition underwent excision of the lesion of the spermatic cord (55520). There was mild systemic disease (P2). In this case, a spermatic cord lipoma was found upon surgery and was therefore removed. The anesthesia (00830) was for hernia repairs in lower abdomen; not otherwise specified.

Case 56: Intraperitoneal procedure in the upper abdomen, including laparoscopy

- Discharge Summary
- Discharge Diagnosis: Hyperglycemia, cholelithiasis, obstructive sleep apnea, insulin-dependent diabetes mellitus, and cholecystitis
- Procedure: Laparoscopic cholecystectomy
- Anesthesia: General endotracheal; difficult intubation
- Anesthesiologist personally provided the general endotracheal anesthesia for the case (PS III)
- Anesthesia time: 2.05 hours
- History of Present Illness
- Patient is a 48-year-old woman suffering from morbid obesity, also known to suffer from diabetes and obstructive sleep apnea. She has been evaluated in the bariatric surgical center for placement of a lap band. During this evaluation, evidence of cholelithiasis was found, and it was decided that removal of the gallbladder prior to placement of the band would be prudent. The patient was scheduled to undergo her outpatient procedure on Thursday; however, at a blood glucose check on Wednesday morning, the patient was noted to be hyperglycemic, as her blood sugar was 453. She was admitted to the hospital on Wednesday for treatment of her hyperglycemia.
- Hospital Course of Treatment
- Patient was admitted to the hospital. Dr. placed her on an insulin drip in an attempt to control the hyperglycemia. Her sugars did slowly come down to between 110 and 130. The patient was placed on the CPAP machine at night for the management of sleep apnea. On the next day, she was then taken to the operating room, where she underwent her laparoscopic cholecystectomy. She was noted to be difficult intubation the procedure. There were some indications of chronic cholecystitis, mild edema, and adhesions of omentum around the gallbladder. She tolerated it without much difficulty, recovered in the recovery area, and was returned to the floor. Her blood sugar postprocedural was noted to be 240. She was started back on sliding scale insulin. She continued to do well and was felt to be stable for discharge following the procedure.
- Discharge Instructions
- Patient will return to the Medifast diet and continue monitoring the blood glucose levels. Patient will follow up with Dr. the surgeon and Dr. Endocrinologist next week. We will determine if we will proceed with her lap band at that time. She may shower and needs to keep her wounds clean and dry. No heavy lifting. No driving on narcotic pain medicines. She needs to continue with her CPAP machine and continue to monitor her sugars.

Codes

47562, 99223, 31500-22, 94660, K80.10, E11.65, G47.33, K66.0, E66.01, Z79.4

Overall anesthesiology code for the case for the billing anesthesiologist

00790-AA-P3

Units calculation=16.2

Clinical viewpoint

The patient has insulin-dependent diabetes mellitus with hyperglycemia (E11.65) which was controlled in the hospital (99223). She in addition has obstructive sleep apnea (G47.33) requiring placement on a CPAP machine for continuous positive airway pressure (CPAP) ventilation (94660) in the hospital. The patient also had morbid (severe) obesity due to excess calories (E66.01). For cholelithiasis and chronic cholecystitis (K80.10), she underwent a laparoscopic cholecystectomy (47562). There were peritoneal adhesions (K66.0) around the omentum near the gallbladder. The intubation was a difficult intubation and required increased procedural services (31500-22). In this case, it is important to note that the intubation required for anesthesia was difficult.

Case 57: Intraperitoneal procedure in the upper abdomen, including laparoscopy; Page gastric restrictive for morbid obesity

- Surgery Consultation
- Visit for evacuation of elective surgical weight loss methods
- History of Present Illness
- Patient has been previously seen in my office for evaluation for a potential elective surgical weight loss procedure. The patient is a 32-year-old female with a BMI of 42.7. Her current weight is 241, and her height is 5'3". She is currently struggling with hypertension and shortness of breath related to her morbid obesity. She also has a great personal motivation to want to lose weight as she states she'd like to increase her energy level and be able to improve her self-image.
- Patient has participated in many weight loss programs over the years, but always gains back more weight than she has lost. She states she lost 100 pounds on Redux but gained it all back plus. She also has tried Weight Watchers, Atkins, Slim Fast, Dexatrim, and Resistant Starch, with varying degrees of success.
- Past Medical History
    - Positive for hypertension and shortness of breath
    - Past Surgical History
    - Cholecystectomy, 1999
    - Psychological History
    - Mild depression
    - Social History
    - Patient is unmarried. Works as administrative assistant. She drinks socially and does not smoke.
    - Family History
    - Obesity and heart disease—mother and father
    - Current Medications
    - Topamax 100 mg twice daily (migraines), Zoloft 100 mg twice daily, multivitamin
    - Allergies
    - No known drug allergies
    - Review of Systems
    - Shortness of breath as discussed above, all others negative
- Examination
    - Patient is alert and oriented X 3, in no acute distress.
    - HEENT: Normocephalic, atraumatic. Extraocular muscles are intact. Anicteric sclerae.
    - Chest: Chest is clear to auscultation bilaterally. Cardiovascular is normal sinus rhythm.

    - Abdomen: The abdomen is obese, soft, non-tender, and non distended.
    - Extremities: Extremities show no edema, clubbing, or cyanosis.
- Assessment and Plan
    - Patient is interested in elective surgical weight loss via the lap band procedure. She will be asking for a letter of medical necessity from her primary care physician. We will schedule appointments with our nutritionist and social worker as well and will submit all information once complete to her insurance company for approval.
- Procedure: Lap band for elective surgical weight loss
- Anesthesia: General endotracheal
- Anesthesiologist provided the general endotracheal anesthesia for the case directing one CRNA (PS III)
- Anesthesia time: 2.25 hours

Codes

43770, 99244, E66.01, I10, R06.02, Z68.41, Z82.49, Z84.89

Overall anesthesiology code for the case for the billing anesthesiologist

00797-QY-P3

Overall anesthesiology code for the billing CRNA

00797-QX-P3

Units calculation=21.0

Clinical viewpoint

The anesthesia (00797) was for intraperitoneal procedures in upper abdomen including laparoscopy; gastric restrictive procedure (43770) for morbid obesity (E66.01). The laparoscopic gastric restrictive procedure included placement of adjustable gastric restrictive device (e.g. gastric band and subcutaneous port components. For a patient with morbid obesity, Body Mass Index (BMI) (Z68.41) should be medically coded for.

Case 58: Nerves, muscles, tendons, fascia, and bursae of the shoulder and axilla

- Postoperative Diagnosis: Left breast cancer (DCIS)
- Procedures Performed: Left segmental mastectomy
- Left axillary sentinel node biopsy
- Surgeon: Dr. Optum
- Anesthesia: General endotracheal (PS III)
- Anesthesia time: 4.07 hours
- Anesthesiologist provided the anesthesia for the case while directing 4 CRNAs
- Estimated Blood Loss: Minimal
- Description of Procedure: The patient was placed supine on the operating table. General anesthesia was induced. An incision was made in the left axillary skin and deepened through the subcutaneous tissues into the axillary fat pad. The first lymph node was removed and was not blue. Ex vivo had counts in the 53 range. It was submitted as axillary lymph node #1. The second node was identified by the gamma counter and was also removed clipping lymphatics with Hemoclips and ex vivo. The node had counts in the range of 3. That was submitted as lymph node #2. There were additional counts in the axilla, and a third node was dissected out and this node was indeed stained blue. It was removed and submitted as lymph node #3 and its counts were much stronger in the range of 270. The axilla was irrigated with saline. Hemostasis was checked and found to be complete. The tissues were closed with 3-0 Vicryl and running 4-0 Monocryl subcuticular. Dr. X from pathology called and advised that there was a total of 5 sentinel nodes in the specimens and that all were negative for malignancy.
- A transverse curvilinear incision was then made overlying the palpable mass in the superior aspect of the left breast. Dissection was deepened through the subcutaneous tissues. The mass was dissected out with a margin around it using electrocautery and removed from the patient. The superior margin was marked with a single silk stitch. The lateral margin was marked with 2 silk stitches and the inferior margin was marked with 3 silk stitches. I personally took the specimen out to the pathologist and described the patient and the situation. After scrubbing back in, the wound was then irrigated with saline. Hemostasis was confirmed. There was no significant residual breast tissue superiorly, and the dissection along the deep aspect was down to the pectoralis muscle. Medial, lateral, and inferior marginal biopsies were than taken with scissors, and the new true margin was marked with blue ink and these margins were submitted individually for marginal biopsies for the frozen section. The medial and inferior wounds were negative. The lateral one had some residual DCIS, and therefore additional lateral margin was harvested and marked accordingly. The superior

aspect of this margin was identified with a 4-0 nylon stitch, and this sample was immediately taken to pathology. They reported back later and confirmed that there was no residual cancer in this final margin. Again, the wound was irrigated. Hemostasis was completed with electrocautery. There was excellent hemostasis. A drain was not deemed to be necessary. The wound was closed with 3-0 Vicryl to the subcutaneous tissue and running 4-0 Monocryl subcuticular in the skin. Dressings were applied and the procedure completed. Sponge, needle, and instrument counts reported as correct. The patient tolerated the procedure well. She was awakened, extubated, and taken to recovery room to recovery room in satisfactory condition.

- Operative Findings
- There were 3 sentinel nodes that were all negative for malignancy. The patient had a mass in the superior aspect of the left breast that was widely excised as a segmental mastectomy, positive for intraductal carcinoma in situ. Marginal biopsies were taken, and the lateral one had residual DCIS. At that point, an additional marginal biopsy was taken and was negative.

Codes

19301, 38525, 88309, D05.12

Overall anesthesiology code for the case for the billing anesthesiologist

01610-QK-P3

Overall anesthesiology code for the case for the billing CRNA

01610-QX-P3

Units calculation= 22.28

Clinical viewpoint

The patient has intraductal carcinoma in situ of the left breast (D05.12) and underwent left segmental mastectomy (19301) and left axillary sentinel node biopsy (38525). 3 sentinel lymph nodes were removed and sent to pathology as specimens (88309). The biopsy or excision were of open, deep axillary nodes. The anesthesia (01610) is for all procedures on nerves, muscles, tendons, fascia, and bursae of shoulder and axilla.

Case 59: Intraperitoneal procedure in the upper abdomen, including laparoscopy

- Postoperative diagnosis: Recurrent diverticular disease in the sigmoid colon
- Procedures Performed: Laparoscopic sigmoid resection
- Laparoscopic mobilization of the splenic flexure
- Flexible sigmoidoscopy at the completion of the anastomosis to verify patency
- Surgeon: Dr. Optum
- Anesthesia: General endotracheal and local and postoperative pain pump inserted and implanted intra-arterially
- Anesthesiologist personally provided the general endotracheal anesthesia for the case (PS III)
- The anesthesiologist started the anesthesia at the beginning of the case and completed the anesthesia post-operatively when the pain pump was inserted
- Anesthesia time: 2.25 hours
- Specimens received: Sigmoid colon—segment measuring approximately 15 to 18 inches
- Blood loss: 50 ml
- Patient Disposition: Recovery room
- Description of Procedure: The patient was brought into the OR. General anesthesia was induced without difficulty. Opt view technique was used in the abdominal cavity via a right lateral abdominal wall. Pneumoperitoneum was established without any complications. The patient had obvious adhesions to the left lateral pelvic sidewall from diverticular disease. We (surgeons) were able to identify the site of involvement. We took down the entire splenic flexure without injury to the spleen or bleeding from the spleen and mobilization of the omentum to the distal transverse colon. We were able to completely mobilize the left colon without difficulty, bleeding, or injury to any surrounding structures. We then placed a small incision in the suprapubic midline for the wound retractor. This was placed in the standard fashion without complication. We were able to eviscerate the sigmoid colon. We transacted proximally using a GIA 75 mm stapler in the descending colon. We transacted distally at the recto-sigmoid junction on the rectal side using a green contour stapler. We took the mesentery of the colon using the Harmonic Ace device. No significant bleeding or complications. Segment was sent off the table. Proximal bowel was palpable and healthy. No obvious diverticular disease. Distal bowel was rectum. No diverticular disease present in the rectum as noted. We the sized from below using a 25 then a 29-mm sizer. We selected a 29 mm EEA stapler. On the proximal bowel, I removed the staple line and placed my anvil and placed a purse string after placement of the anvil in the end fashion of the colon. From below, we brought the EEA stapler into the staple line and brought the spike out from the EEA

stapler on the anterior rectal surface in order to perform our end-to-side anastomosis. The EEA stapler was fired in standard fashion. Two doughnuts were identified in the black table confirming a normal anastomosis was performed. We then clamped the colon proximally and performed a flexible sigmoidoscopy, hyper inflating the colon. Noting that there was no intraluminal bleeding, the anastomosis was widely patent. There was no bubble leak identified, negative provocative leak test intra-abdominally with the anastomosis submerged in saline. I then decompressed the colon lumen and removed the scope. I then irrigated the abdominal cavity, confirmed all counts were correct, placed 10 ml of fibrin glue around the anastomosis, and removed the wound retractor. The patient tolerated the procedure well and was taken to recovery.

Codes

44204+44213, 45330, 88309, K57.30

Overall anesthesiology code for the case for the billing anesthesiologist

00790-AA-P3, 36260

Units calculation= 17.0

Clinical viewpoint

The patient has diverticular disease in the sigmoid colon (K57.30) without perforation, abscess, or bleeding. The patient underwent laparoscopy, surgical, colectomy, partial with anastomosis with surgical, mobilization (take-down) of splenic flexure performed in conjunction with partial colectomy (44204+44213). The patient also received flexible sigmoidoscopy, diagnostic, including the collection of specimen(s) by brushing or washing, when performed (45330). The specimen of segmental sigmoid colon (88309) measuring 15 to 18 inches was sent to pathology. The anesthesia (00790) was for intraperitoneal procedures in upper abdomen including laparoscopy; not otherwise specified. In this case, for anesthesia after the operation, a pain pump was inserted and implanted intra-arterially postoperatively (36260). The code for insertion of the pain pump is included in the Overall anesthesiology code for the case for the billing anesthesiologist.

Case 60: Access to the central venous circulation

- Postoperative Diagnosis: Severe chronic obstructive pulmonary disease
- Respiratory failure
- Procedure Performed: Placement of right subclavian triple lumen central line
- Anesthesia: Local Xylocaine
- Anesthesiologist personally performed the local anesthesia for the case (PS IV)
- Anesthesia time (for the procedure): 35 minutes
- Critical care time: 60 minutes
- Blood Loss: Minimal
- Indications Referral from Dr. Q requesting central line placement. This 54-year-old male patient in severe respiratory failure is on mechanical ventilation. This patient currently requires multiple IV drips, and the triple lumen catheter is to assist with these multiple IVs.
- Description of Procedure
- Patient is in his bed in the ICU, currently being mechanically ventilated. The right side of the neck was prepped and draped in a sterile fashion. Single-needle stick aspiration of the right subclavian vein was accomplished without difficulty, and the guide wire was advanced. The dilator was advanced over the wire. The triple-lumen catheter was cannulated over the wire, and the wire was removed. No PVCs were encountered during the procedure. All three ports to the catheter were aspirated and flushed blood easily, and they were all flushed with normal saline. The catheter was anchored to the chest wall with a butterfly syringe using 3-0 silk suture. Betadine ointment and sterile Op-Site dressing were applied. Stat upright chest x-ray was obtained at the completion of the procedure, and final results showed good catheter placement. Patient seemed to tolerate the procedure well.

Codes

36561, 99291, 31500, J2001, J44.9, J96.90

Overall anesthesiology code for the case for the billing anesthesiologist

36561

Note that the anesthesia was local anesthesia in this case which is bundled with the anesthesia code

Clinical viewpoint

The patient is intubated (31500) on mechanical ventilation in the ICU (99291). He underwent placement of right subclavian triple lumen central line with subcutaneous port (36561) under Local anesthesia. The patient has severe chronic pulmonary disease (J44.9) and respiratory failure (J96.90). He has severe systemic disease that is a constant threat to life (PS IV). In this case, Local anesthesia with Xylocaine is bundled with the procedure. The local anesthesia injection was of lidocaine HCL, 10 mg (J2001) for intravenous infusion.

Case 61: Upper gastro-intestinal endoscopic procedure, endoscope introduced proximal to the duodenum

- Postoperative Diagnosis:
- Heartburn
- Diverticulosis of the colon
- Internal hemorrhoids
- Possible short segment Barrett esophagus
- Procedure Performed:
- Colonoscopy with internal hemorrhoid banding x 1
- Flexible esophagogastroduodenoscopy with biopsies
- Surgeon:
- Dr. Optum
- Anesthesia:
- MAC anesthesia with topical for EGD in pharynx
- Anesthesiologist performed the monitored anesthesia care (MAC) service for the case while directing one CRNA (PS III)
- Anesthesia time: 1.50 hours
- Estimated Blood Loss:
- Minimal
- Description of Procedure:
- The flexible Olympus upper GI endoscope was passed through the bite block into the posterior pharynx. The esophageal orifice was identified and cannulated. Insufflation, irrigation, and suction were utilized appropriately, and representative photographs were taken. The scope was advanced down the esophagus into the stomach, past pylorus into the duodenum, brought back into the stomach, retroflexed on itself. Biopsies were taken with cold biopsy forceps of the antral mucosa for urease testing and of the distal esophagus for histopathology analysis and no significant ongoing hemorrhage ensued. The gas suctioned, scope removed slowly and carefully, and this portion of the procedure was terminated.
- Olympus colonoscope was inserted into the anal canal and advanced into the rectum. The scope was advanced into the recto sigmoid junction, negotiated through a very loopy, redundant sigmoid colon into the descending colon. I was able to get past the splenic flexure. I was able to get past the transverse colon and the hepatic flexure into the ascending colon, ultimately past the ileocecal valve into the cecum.
- A digital rectal exam was performed and then I proceeded to perform band ligation with single prominent internal hemorrhoid, and the Olympus upper GI endoscope was fitted with the multiband ligator as per standard routine. The

hemorrhoid was suctioned and the band deployed. The band was adequately placed and the other surrounding hemorrhoids did not appear to be amenable to band ligation as they were much smaller and less prominent. The air was suctioned and the scope removed.

- Findings:
- The patient had normal laryngeal and posterior pharyngeal structures. The esophageal orifice was normal, proximal and middle esophagus normal. The GE junction was situated approximately 40 cm from the incisors. There was certainly some irregularity at the GE junction and a couple of tiny islands of gastric-type mucosa suggesting the presence of a short segment Barrett esophagus.
- The length was certainly only a few millimeters. No evidence of strictures, rings, diverticula, or significant esophagitis was seen. No significant hiatal hernia was appreciated. No polyps or carcinoma. The gastric lumen distended normally. There were no ulcers, no polyps, and no evidence of malignancy. The cardia, fundus, body, antrum, and prepyloric areas were all normal. The pylorus was patent and normal. The duodenal bulb, second, third, and fourth portions, of the duodenum were normal. A random biopsy of the antral mucosa was obtained for urease testing, and biopsies of the distal esophagus were obtained to assess for the presence of Barrett metaplasia.
- Colonoscopy revealed fairly good bowel prep, although areas of the cecum and ascending colon were a bit under-prepped and probably future bowel prep should be a bit more aggressive. In any event, the patient does have some scattered medium mouthed diverticula in the left colon. No evidence of diverticulitis or strictures was seen. No polyps were seen. No evidence of carcinoma was seen. The patient had an exceedingly redundant sigmoid colon with the entire length of the colonoscope inserted by about the mid transverse colon quite a lot of manipulation and counter pressure to the abdominal wall again access to the cecum, which was ultimately successful but required a lot of effort. The patient does have internal hemorrhoids, which were not bleeding. There was one in particular that appeared more anteriorly situated. It appeared to be larger than the rest and mildly inflamed and I chose that for internal bleeding; utilizing the multiband ligator, I placed a single band on that particular hemorrhoid without incident.

Codes

45398, 43239-59-53, 88305, 88305+88314, K64.8, K57.30, R12, K22.70

Overall anesthesiology code for the case for the billing anesthesiologist

00731-QS-QY-P3

Overall anesthesiology code for the case for the billing CRNA

00731-QS-QX-P3

Units calculation=12.0

Clinical viewpoint

The patient is being treated for heartburn (R12), diverticulosis of colon (K57.30), internal hemorrhoids (K64.8), and possible short segment Barrett esophagus (K22.70). The patient underwent flexible esophagogastroduodenoscopy, transoral, diagnostic with biopsy, single or multiple (43239-59-53) and flexible colonoscopy, diagnostic with band ligation(s) (e.g., hemorrhoids) with specimens sent to pathology for histopathology analysis (+88314) of stomach biopsy (88305) and esophagus biopsy (88305) for presence of Barrett metaplasia. The anesthesia (00731) is for upper gastrointestinal procedures, endoscope introduced proximal to duodenum. The anesthesia was monitored anesthesia care (MAC) service (QS).

Case 62: Integumentary system on the extremities, anterior trunk, and perineum

- Date of Procedure: XX/XX/XXXX
- Postoperative Diagnosis: Abscess, left leg, positive for MRSA
- Procedure Performed: Incision and drainage left leg
- Surgeon: Dr. Optum
- Anesthesia: Regional block with moderate sedation
- Anesthesiologist personally provided the regional anesthesia for the case (PS III)
- Anesthesia time: 35 minutes
- Estimated Blood Loss: Less than 25 ml
- Description of Procedure: The patient was brought into the operating room. The regional block had been previously administered in the holding area. Anesthesia administered the moderate sedation. The skin was incised sharply with a scalpel over the fluctuant mass in the anteromedial left leg. Copious amount of purulence was drained; this was suctioned. The wound was probed and the fibrous bands were broken up. Hemostasis was achieved with electrocautery. The wound was then packed with Betadine-soaked gauze. A dry dressing was placed around this followed by an Ace wrap. The patient tolerated the procedure well. He was transported to the recovery area in stable condition.
- Findings: Pathology reports MRSA in the purulent drainage sent and cultured. Start patient on Clindamycin 600 mg IV.

Codes

10061, 88304, L02.416, B95.62

Overall anesthesiology code for the case for the billing anesthesiologist

00400-AA-P3

Units calculation= 6.33

Clinical viewpoint

The patient underwent Incision and drainage of a complicated abscess of the leg (10061) and purulent drainage sent to pathology (88304). The cutaneous abscess of the lower limb (L02.416) had MRSA in the purulent drainage (B95.62). The anesthesia is for procedures on the integumentary system on the extremities, anterior trunk, and perineum; not otherwise specified (00400). The procedure was a major procedure requiring regional block with moderate sedation. Regional block is coded as an anesthesiology code, as it is one of the four types of anesthesia (General, regional, monitored anesthesia care, and local). Local anesthesia is bundled with the procedure.

Case 63: Vascular shunt, or shunt revision, any type (e.g., dialysis); injection, anesthetic agent, suprascapular nerve

- Date of Operation: XX/XX/XXXX
- Postoperative Diagnosis: End-stage renal disease with need for dialysis access. Staged right brachiobasilic arteriovenous fistula creation.
- Procedure Performed: Transposition right brachiobasilic AV fistula in the subcutaneous tunnel—completion of procedure started XX/XX/XXXX
- Surgeon: Dr. Optum
- Anesthesia: Supraclavicular block, followed by general endotracheal anesthesia
- Anesthesiologist personally provided the supraclavicular block followed by general endotracheal anesthesia
- The anesthesiologist started the anesthesia with the supraclavicular block and completed the anesthesia post-operatively in the recovery room
- Anesthesia time: 3.35 hours
- Indications: This 52-year-old female end-stage renal disease patient is in need of permanent dialysis access. This patient currently requires hemodialysis using a temporary dialysis catheter. At this time, the second and final phase of a staged right brachiobasilic arteriovenous fistula creation will be completed.
- Estimated blood loss: Minimal
- Description of Procedure: It ultimately became necessary to induce general anesthesia in this patient. The entire procedure was done under 2.5X loop magnification. The vein was exposed with a longitudinal incision over the inner aspect of the right upper arm, lengthening the incision in stepwise fashion, bringing the vein into view from the elbow to the axilla. The vein was then elevated by taking branches between 4-0 silk ties and baby Hem clips. The larger branches were doubly tied on the vein side. The vein was now much more mobile. A pocket was developed in the subcutaneous tissues out laterally over the biceps muscle, elevating the skin and fat layer up and away from the underlying fascia. The vein was positioned out over the biceps muscle, and the tissues were then reapproximated down over the vein with interrupted 3-0 Vicryl, being sure not the put any undue pressure on the vein. A good strong thrill was maintained throughout. The wound was then irrigated with saline. The subcutaneous tissue was closed with 3-0 Vicryl. Skin was closed with simple and vertical mattress sutures of 4-0 nylon. Dressings were applied as well as an arm board and the procedure completed. Sponge, needle, and instrument counts reported as correct. Patient tolerated the procedure well. She was awakened, extubated, and taken to recovery room in satisfactory condition.

Codes

36819-RT,58, N18.6, Z99.2

Overall anesthesiology code for the case for the billing anesthesiologist

01844-AA-P3, 64418

Units calculation= 20.4

Clinical viewpoint

The patient underwent arteriovenous anastomosis by upper arm basilica transposition (36819) for end-stage renal disease (N18.6) requiring dialysis access (Z99.2). The anesthesia (01844) was for vascular shunt, or shunt revision, any type (e.g. dialysis). Supraclavicular block (64418), a nerve block which counts as regional anesthesia was in addition performed prior to the general endotracheal anesthesia and counts as an anesthesiology code.

Case 64: Integumentary system, muscles, and nerves of the head, neck, and posterior trunk

- Date of Procedure: X/XX/XXXX
- Postoperative Diagnosis: Malignant melanoma, chest (1 cm)
- Surgeon: Dr. Optum
- Anesthesia: General endotracheal
- Anesthesiologist personally provided general endotracheal anesthesia (PS IV)
- Anesthesia time: 1.87 hours
- Procedure: Excision of skin lesion of chest wall
- Description of Procedure: The mid-cheek was prepped and draped in sterile fashion, and cleaned with Betadine solution. A margin of 2 cm laterally and medially around the lesion site was taken in addition to the 1 cm lesion. The incision was carried down to the muscle fascia, which was included in the specimen. Bleeding was controlled by electrocautery, and we closed the defect with running subcuticular 4-0 Vicryl using layered closure. Steri-strips and a sterile bandage were applied. The patient tolerated the procedure well.
- Operative Findings: Pathology determined the lesion was malignant melanoma. Margins were clean and it does not appear that additional treatment is required at this time. Appropriate counseling on sun protection and the other risk factors and preventive measures provided.

Codes

11606, 12032-59, C43.59

Overall anesthesiology code

00300-AA-P4

Units calculation= 14.48

Clinical viewpoint

The patient has malignant melanoma of the chest (C43.59) and underwent excision of malignant skin lesion of the chest wall with 2 cm margins for a 1 cm lesion size for a total excised diameter of 5 cm (11606) with repair, intermediate, wounds of scalp, axillae, trunk and/or extremities (excluding hands and feet); 2.6 cm to 7.5 cm for the layered closure. The anesthesia (00300) was for all procedures on the integumentary system, muscles and nerves of head, neck, and posterior trunk, not otherwise specified. The patient has severe systemic disease, malignant melanoma which is a constant threat to life (P4).

Case 65: Upper gastrointestinal endoscopic procedures, endoscope introduced proximal to the duodenum

- Date of Procedure: XX/XX/XXXX
- Postoperative Diagnosis: Abdominal pain, cystic lesions of pancreas, suspicious for branchial intraductal papillary mucinous neoplasm
- Surgeon: Dr. Optum
- Anesthesia: Monitored anesthesia care (MAC) service
- Anesthesiologist personally provided the monitored anesthesia care (MAC) service (PS II)
- Anesthesia time: 55 minutes
- Procedure: Upper endoscopic ultrasound
- Description of Procedure: After obtaining informed consent the endoscope was passed under vision. Throughout the procedure, the patient's blood pressure, pulse, and oxygen saturation were monitored continuously. The endoscopic with transducer was introduced through the mouth and advanced to the second part of the duodenum. Findings are detailed below. The upper EUS was accomplished without difficulty. The patient tolerated the procedure well.
- Endosonographic Findings: An anechoic lesion suggestive of a cyst was identified in the pancreatic head. The lesion measured 4 mm by 3 mm. There was no associated mass.
- An anechoic lesion suggestive of a cyst was identified in the pancreatic neck. The lesion measured 9 mm by 8 mm. There was no associated mass. There was no internal debris within the fluid-filled cavity.
- An anechoic lesion suggestive of a cyst was identified in the pancreatic body. The lesion measured 7 mm by 6 mm. There was no associated mass. There was no internal debris within the fluid-filled cavity.
- The celiac axis including lymph nodes was unremarkable. The examined portion of the left lobe of the liver and the gastrohepatic ligament were evaluated and found to be without abnormalities.
- The pancreas was examined and the parenchyma demonstrated three cystic lesions as above. The main pancreatic duct measured 1.7 mm in the head, 1.1 mm in the body, and 1.0 mm in the tail. The ampulla was normal endoscopically and endosonographically. The bile duct ranged in size from 1.9 mm to 2.4 mm in size and was normal in appearance. The gallbladder was normal in appearance.
- Overall Impression: A 4 mm by 3 mm cystic lesion was seen in the pancreatic head. Tissue has not been obtained. However, the endosonographic appearance is highly suspicious for a branched intraductal papillary mucinous neoplasm.
- A 9 mm by 8 mm cystic lesion was seen in the pancreatic neck. Tissue has not been obtained. However, the endosonographic appearance is highly suspicious for branched intraductal papillary mucinous neoplasm.

- A 7 mm by 6 mm cystic lesion was seen in the pancreatic body. Tissue has not been obtained. However, the endosonographic appearance is highly suspicious of for branched intraductal papillary mucinous neoplasm.

Codes

43237, K86.2

Overall anesthesiology code for the case for the billing anesthesiologist

00731-AA-QS-P2

Units calculation=8.67

Clinical viewpoint

The patient has cysts of the pancreas (K86.2) and underwent esophagogastroduodenoscopy, flexible, transoral; with endoscopic ultrasound examination limited to esophagus, stomach or duodenum, and adjacent structures (43237). The anesthesia (00731) is for upper gastrointestinal endoscopic procedures, endoscope introduced proximal to duodenum. Note that the anesthesia is monitored anesthesia care (MAC) service (QS).

Case 66: Extraperitoneal procedures in the lower abdomen, including urinary tract; adrenalectomy

- Postoperative Diagnosis: Adrenal mass, right sided
- Umbilical hernia
- Procedure Performed: Umbilical hernia repair
- Anesthesia: General endotracheal
- Anesthesiologist personally provided the general endotracheal anesthesia for the case while directing 5 CRNAs (PS IV)
- Anesthesia time: 2.05 hours
- Indications: This is a 48-year-old patient with a 4.2 cm diameter mass in his right adrenal gland and umbilical hernia. Alternative of fully laparoscopic are open surgery or simply watching the adrenal lesion for further treatment in the future. Patient has decided to pursue removal of the lesion and repair the umbilical hernia at the time.
- Description of Procedure:
- An incision was made from just above the umbilicus, about 5.5 cm in diameter. The umbilical hernia was taken down. An 11-mm trocar was placed in the midline, superior to the Gel Port and a 5-mm trocar placed in the midaxillary line below the costal margin. A liver retractor was placed.
- The colon was reflected medially by incising the white line of Toldt. The liver attachments to the adrenal kidney were divided, and the liver was reflected superiorly. The vena cava identified. The main renal vein was identified. Coming superior to the main renal vein, staying right on the vena cava, all small vessels were clipped and then divided. Coming along the superior pole of the kidney, the tumor was dissected free from the top of the kidney with clips and Bovie. The harmonic scalpel was utilized superiorly and laterally. Posterior attachments were divided between clips and once the whole adrenal was mobilized, the adrenal vein and one large adrenal artery were noted, doubly clipped, and divided. The specimen was placed in a collection bag and removed intact. Hemostasis was excellent.
- The umbilical hernia had been completely taken down. The edges were freshened up. #1 Vicryl was utilized to close the incision and 2-0 Vicryl was used to close the fascia of the trocar. The skin closed with clips. The patient tolerated the procedure well. All sponge and instrument counts were correct. The patient was awakened, extubated, and returned to recovery room in satisfactory condition.

Codes

60545, 49587-59, 12032-51, 88307, E27.8, K42.9

Overall anesthesiology code for the case for the billing anesthesiologist

00866-AD-P4

Overall anesthesiologist code for the case for the billing CRNA

00866-QX-P4

Units calculation= 20.2

Clinical viewpoint

The patient underwent adrenalectomy with excision of adjacent retroperitoneal tumor (60545) and incarcerated umbilical hernia repair (49587-59) for right-sided adrenal mass (E27.8) and umbilical hernia (K42.9). The anesthesia is for extra peritoneal procedures in lower abdomen, including urinary tract; adrenalectomy. Note that the anesthesiologist directed 5 CRNAs (AD) and the CRNA service was with medical direction by a physician (QX).

Case 67: Upper gastrointestinal endoscopic procedures, endoscope introduced proximal to duodenum

- Postoperative Diagnosis: ALS, dysphagia
- Procedure Performed: Percutaneous endoscopic gastrostomy tube placement
- Anesthesia: General endotracheal
- Anesthesiologist personally provided the general endotracheal anesthesia for the case (PS III)
- Anesthesia time: 42 minutes
- Indications: Patient is a 46-year-old male requiring PEG tube placement due to dysphagia secondary to ALS. Placement of the tube was requested by the patient's neurologist.
- Description of Procedure: The flexible endoscope was advanced through the oropharynx, past the epiglottis, and into the upper esophagus. It was then advanced into the stomach, which was partially insufflated with air. The pyloris was identified and intubated, and we surveyed the second portion of the duodenum and the duodenal sweep. These were each normal. The stomach was normal on retroflexed view. There was no hiatal hernia. The gastric mucosa appeared normal. The patient's stomach was then fully insufflated with air until the rugae were flattened. The local needle was then passed through the patient's skin through his abdominal wall and directly into the stomach. There was no air that was found by aspiration along this route, and it was noted to enter easily into the patient's abdomen. This was then replaced by the introducer needle and was grasped with the endoscope and was withdrawn through the patient's mouth. A PEG tube was then attached to the guidewire and then returned in an ante grade fashion through the patient's esophagus and out the gastric wall through a stab incision. The endoscope was re-advanced into the stomach and the stomach was surveyed. There was no bleeding that was seen. The PEG tube was withdrawn until it reached a depth of 3 cm. At depth of 3 cm, it was seen not to blanch the gastric mucosa, yet not appear to be too loose. This appropriate placement for the PEG tube. The endoscope was then withdrawn. The scope was then withdrawn after desufflating the stomach, and the procedure terminated. The patient tolerated the procedure well and was taken to the recovery room in stable condition.

Codes

43246, R13.10, G12.21

Overall anesthesiology code for the case for the billing CRNA

00731-AA-P3

Units calculation=8.8

Clinical viewpoint

The patient underwent esophagogastroduodenoscopy, flexible, trans oral; with directed placement of percutaneous gastrostomy tube (43246) for dysphagia (R13.10) secondary to amyotrophic lateral sclerosis (ALS) (G12.21). The anesthesia (00731) is for upper gastrointestinal endoscopic procedures, endoscope introduced proximal to duodenum.

Case 68: Anorectal

- Postoperative Diagnosis: Anal condyloma
- Procedure Performed: Excision and cautery destruction of anal condyloma
- Surgeon: Dr. Optum
- Anesthesia: Monitored anesthesia care
- Anesthesia time: 35 minutes
- 0.5% Marcaine with epinephrine locally
- Anesthesiologist provided the monitored anesthesia care service for the case directing one CRNA (PS II)
- Details of Procedure: The patient was brought to the operative suite, identified, placed in the prone jackknife position, and anesthesia was induced. A Betadine prep was carried out. The areas were grasped, pulled up and excised at their bases and the mucosa with a knife. Specimens were sent for pathology. The base of the lesion was then cauterized with the needle-tipped cautery. Multiple areas externally and into the internal canal were removed and cauterized.
- There were no immediate complications. Sterile dressing was placed over the wounds. He tolerated the procedure well and was taken to the recovery area in satisfactory condition.
- Surgical Findings: There were multiple anal condyloma externally and some in the internal anal canal up to the dentate line. These were all excised and the base destroyed with the cautery.

Codes

46924, 88304, A63.0

Overall anesthesiology code for the case for the billing anesthesiologist

00902-QY-QS-P2

Overall anesthesiology code for case for the billing CRNA

00902-QX-QS-P2

Units calculation= 7.33

Clinical viewpoint

The patient underwent Destruction of lesion(s), anus (e.g. condyloma, papilloma, molluscum contagiosum, herpetic vesicle), extensive (e.g. laser surgery, electro surgery, cryosurgery, chemosurgery), as there were multiple anal condyloma externally (A63.0) and some in the internal anal canal up to the dentate line. The specimen was sent to pathology (88304). The anesthesia (00902) is for; anorectal procedure. The anesthesiologist (QY) directed one CRNA (QX) for this monitored anesthesia care service (QS).

Case 69: Lower intestinal endoscopic procedure, endoscope introduced distal to the duodenum

- Date of Service: XX/XX/XXXX
- Chief Complaint: Pain in abdomen
- History of Present Illness: Patient is a 58-year-old white female with a past medical history significant for an MI and depression who presents today complaining of sharp, epigastric pain of approximately 2 months duration. The abdominal pain has been gradually worsening over the past 3 weeks. The pain is located in the epigastric region of the abdomen. It does not typically radiate. The pain is not alleviated at rest and is associated with food or eating, although the patient does deal with occasional heartburn as well. Patient denies any abdominal trauma or injury. Patient described a "lump in the throat" with associated dysphagia. She has experienced some nausea with the abdominal pain but has not vomited, and also has had constipation. She endorses blood stools with some bowel movements. The blood is dark red in color and is not bright red. There is sufficient amount of blood to turn the toilet water red. Patient does not know how many times per week she experiences the bleeding. She has not seen a bloody bowel movement in the past week.
- Past Medical History: Well controlled hypertension
- Poorly controlled depression—takes Prozac, but still feels depressed
- Hospitalizations: MI, 2008
- Surgeries/procedures: Cardiac catheterization, 2008
- Medications: Aspirin 81 mg po qd since her MI
- Metoprolol 100 mg po qd
- Prozac 20 mg po qd; started 6 months ago
- NKDA
- Family History: Mother died at age 72 of "natural causes"
- Father died at age 78 of AAA
- No known family history of colon cancer
- Social history: Patient is a retired school secretary. She is divorced with 5 children and 3 grandchildren. She sees them regularly but feels sad and alone. Denies use of tobacco, illicit drugs, or alcohol.
- Review of systems: Constitutional—Decreased appetite, 5 lb. weight loss, fatigue
    - Throat—complains of "lump in throat," dysphagia
    - Gastrointestinal—sharp, epigastric pain, bloody stools
    - All others negative
    - Physical exam: Vital signs: Ht 5'3" wt. 160 lbs. HR 80 RR 16 BP 126/78
    - General: Patient is a well-nourished white female in no acute distress
    - Lymph nodes: Nontender, no palpable masses
    - Neck: No masses

    - Cardiovascular: Regular rate and rhythm; normal S1, S2; no murmurs, rubs, or gallops
    - Lungs: Lungs clear to auscultation bilaterally; no wheezes or crackles
    - Abdominal: Abdomen soft and nondistended with no scars or striations
    - No pulsatile masses, no abdominal bruits auscultated
    - Tender to palpation in epigastric region and left upper quadrant; no reflux tenderness; no guarding; Murphy's sign negative
    - Rectal: Hem occult positive
- Diagnostic tests: Hem occult positive stool
- Assessment & Plan
- Problem List: Abdominal pain
- Melena
- Hem occult was positive for blood in the stool. Discussed with patient the need to schedule a colonoscopy to evaluate the colon for presence of polyps or tumors. Also, start Protonix 40 mg po bid to decrease the level of acid in the stomach.
- Procedure performed: Colonoscopy
- Anesthesia: General endotracheal
- Anesthesiologist personally provided the general endotracheal anesthesia for the case (PS II).
- Anesthesia time: 50 minutes

Codes

99254, 45378, R10.9, K92.1

Overall anesthesiology code for the billing anesthesiologist

00812-AA-P2

Clinical viewpoint

The anesthesia (00812) is for lower intestinal endoscopic procedures, endoscope introduced distal to duodenum. The consult is an inpatient consult (99254). The patient underwent colonoscopy (45378), flexible; diagnostic, including collection of specimen(s) by brushing or washing, when performed (separate procedure) to evaluate for the presence of polyps or tumors. Epigastric pain (R10.13) and melena (K92.1) are the diagnoses.

Case 70: Intraperitoneal procedure in the upper abdomen, including laparoscopy

- Date of Procedure: XX/XX/XXXX
- Postoperative Diagnosis: Idiopathic thrombocytopenia, splenomegaly
- Procedure Performed: Splenectomy
- Anesthesia: General
- Anesthesiologist personally provided the general endotracheal anesthesia for the case (PS III)
- Anesthesia time: 4.07 hours
- Operative Findings: The spleen was larger than expected. Possible hypersplenism causing the thrombocytopenia. Splenic pathology will provide additional details. The liver was without obvious masses. The small bowel, colon, and gall bladder were without any obvious abnormalities.
- Description of Procedure: The patient was taken to the operating room. A midline celiotomy incision was made a few centimeters below the xiphoids to an infraumbilical position. The skin was divided with scalpel followed by cautery for the remaining layers. The fascia was elevated and entered with cautery to gain access to the abdomen. The incision was then extended using cautery. The spleen could be visualized at this point, and it was quite large. There were adhesions at the superior pole to the diaphragm that made attempts to move the spleen toward the midline difficult. These adhesions were divided with cautery. The spleen was pulled down and medial to begin the dissection. The inferior pole near the splenorenal ligament was divided with a combination of cautery and clamps with ties. We then took down short gastric, which freed up the superior pole of the spleen. This created the ability to visualize the hilar structures. The remaining vessels were divided using serially applied clamps and either suture ligature or stick ties as appropriate. Separate divisions of the superior and inferior pole vessels were performed. The spleen was then completely removed and passed off the field as the specimen to be sent to pathology. Hemostasis was obtained using additional stick ties where necessary and argon beam cautery on the raw areas of prior spleen to retroperitoneal attachments and the diaphragmatic attachments to the spleen. After hemostasis was obtained, irrigation was performed. The fascia was closed with a double-looped #1 Maxon suture. The subcutaneous tissue was thoroughly irrigated, and the skin closure was performed with staples. Appropriate dressings were applied. The patient tolerated the procedure well and was transported to recovery in stable condition.

Codes

38100, 88305, D69.3, R16.1

Overall anesthesiology code for the billing anesthesiologist

00790-AA-P3

Units calculation= 24.28

Clinical viewpoint

The patient underwent splenectomy, total (separate procedure) (38100) for splenomegaly (R16.1) caused by immune thrombocytopenic purpura (D69.3). The hypersplenism might be causing the thrombocytopenia. The anesthesia (00790) is for intraperitoneal procedures in upper abdomen including laparoscopy; not otherwise specified.

Case 71: Moderate conscious sedation intra-service

- Time 9:30 A.M. to 10:00 A.M.
- Treating physician as the anesthesiologist provided the moderate conscious sedation with a trained observer to assist in the monitoring of the patient's level of consciousness and physiological status and for the surgical procedure for the case. The patient is a healthy 13-year-old female (PS I) who dislocated her shoulder while playing baseball on a team at the baseball field at her leisure. On physical exam, she was found by his physician to have a right shoulder dislocation. A closed treatment of a right shoulder dislocation is performed by the treating physician.

Codes

S43.004A, Y93.64, Y92.320, Y99.8, 23650, 99152, +99153

Clinical viewpoint

30 minutes of moderate conscious sedation (99152, +99153) was provided by the same physician or other qualified health care professional performing the diagnostic or therapeutic service that the sedation supports, requiring the presence of an independent trained observer.

References

The author gratefully acknowledges that the following excellent references were useful in preparing the contents of this book. These references are reputable in the healthcare field, and extremely helpful in preparing for the CANPC™ exam. The readers are recommended to study these resources for preparation of CANPC™ and career enhancement as medical administrators, coders and billers.

AHA Coding Clinic subscriptions for ICD-10-CM/PCS and HCPCS, American Hospital Association, Chicago, IL, 2000-2016

Practicode CPC-A, COC-A, CPC-A ICD-10 Practicums, American Academy of Professional Coders, Salt Lake City, UT, 2014-2016

ICD-10-CM Coding Workbook for General Surgery, Optum360, Salt Lake City, UT, 2016

Maxim Assessment, Maxim Healthcare Services, Columbia, MD, 2016

Healthcare Business Monthly, American Academy of Professional Coders, Salt Lake City, UT, 2016

An Insider's View: Field Avoidance and Special Positioning, American Academy of Professional Coders, Salt Lake City, UT, 2017

Merriam Webster's Medical Desk Dictionary, Merriam-Webster Incorporated, Clifton Park, NY, 2005

CPT Standard 2022

HCPCS Level II Expert 2022

ICD-10-CM 2022

2022 ASA (American Society of Anesthesiologists) Crosswalk®

2022 ASA Relative Value Guide®

2022 National Physician Fee Schedule Relative Value File January Release copyrighted by 2021 American Medical Association and 2022/23 American Dental Association

PFS Relative Value Files 2022

www.cms.gov

About the book

Taking an examination is stressful at the best of times, and the Certified Anesthesia and Pain Management Coder (CANPC™) exam is no exception. The aim of this book is two-fold: to increase the likelihood that the reader will pass the CANPC™ exam and to make the reader a better medical coder upon receiving this credential.

This book goes beyond the mere presentation of the concepts and applications that aid in passing the exam. It focuses on providing insights into the multitude of scenarios that coders face when presented with actual coding cases. The 71 unique cases presented in the book highlight the correct coding method and provide the reader with practice in applying coding principles to actual patient cases. The author's unique formula allows the reader to arrive at the best coding decision for even the most complicated patient circumstances. Every case is also discussed from a clinical viewpoint (a physician's view) to explain the rationale underlying the different coding decisions.

This book is an invaluable asset for anyone working toward a certificate in anesthesia and pain management coding and facing the CANPC™ exam. It will also serve as a useful reference for those already holding this certificate and working in this complicated and challenging anesthesia and pain management coding field. *The book is compliant with the 2022 codebooks ICD-10-CM, CPT, HCPCS II and 2022 ASA Crosswalk(R), and 2022 Relative Value Guide(R)*

About the author

Vino C. Mody Jr. has worked for 15 years at different US and Swedish hospitals. He has coding certificates from the University of Georgia, U.S. Career Institute, and Blackstone Career Institute. He completed CPMA and specialty courses in CANPC, CCVTC, CEDC, COPC, and CGSC from the American Academy of Professional Coders. Vino also has important coding and billing certifications (COC, CPC, CCS, CCS-P, CMC, CANPC, CCVTC, CEDC, COPC, RMC, REMS, CMAA, CBCS, CICP) *. He has worked as a coding instructor and a consultant for eight years in health care institutes and with coding consultants in El Paso, Texas. Currently, he is a CANPC/CCVTC coding lecturer for the El Paso chapter of AAPC. He has an ICD-10-CM/PCS Trainer certificate from AHIMA. He worked in medical administration at Mesa Hills Hospital in El Paso, Texas, directing coding, auditing, transcription, surgery coding, and software improvement.

Vino has ten years of experience in the field of medicine, and an MD from Emory University School of Medicine in Atlanta, Georgia. He did medical internship at Yale-New Haven Hospital and Brown University/Lifespan Hospital.

Vino has a Ph.D. from Karolinska Institutet in Stockholm, Sweden, where he conducted ophthalmology research and taught Optometry for eight years. Vino published 25 original publications and 100 conference abstracts. He won several research grants from industry. Vino obtained his Bachelor's degree in molecular biology from Vanderbilt University in Nashville, Tennessee, graduating Summa Cum Laude, high honors.

Vino enjoys USTA tennis and has played for the Parkview High School Tennis Team in Georgia and the Atlanta Lawn Tennis Association (ALTA) during his academic years in Georgia.

*Acronyms

COC -	Certified Outpatient Coder
CPC -	Certified Professional Coder
CCS-	Certified Coding Specialist
CCS-P -	Certified Coding Specialist-Physician based
CMC-	Certified Medical Coder
CANPC-	Certified Anesthesia and Pain management Coder
CCVTC -	Certified Cardiovascular and Thoracic surgery Coder
CEDC-	Certified Emergency Department Coder
COPC-	Certified Ophthalmology Coder
RMC-	Registered Medical coder
REMS-	Registered Evaluation & Management Specialist
CMAA -	Certified Medical Administrative Assistant
CBCS -	Certified Billing and Coding Specialist
4Med CICP -	Certificate of ICD - 10 - CM Proficiency

Made in the USA
Monee, IL
20 September 2025

26185152R00072